D1376642

Obsessive-compulsive disorder (OCD) is currently the subject of considerable research. This book offers a critical discussion of the most important theories that have been put forward to explain this disorder.

The book includes behavioural/learning accounts (and cognitive-behavioural supplements of these), accounts based on Pavlovian personality theories (such as those by Eysenck, Gray, and Claridge), Pierre Janet's account, cybernetic approaches, psychodynamic approaches, Reed's cognitive-structural account, and biological approaches. Therapeutic approaches to the disorder are also considered, insofar as they are relevant to these theories. An analysis of the concept of OCD is also presented, together with a critique of the existing definitions of the disorder.

This book is unique in both the comprehensiveness and the depth of its coverage of theories of OCD. It also offers an entirely new approach to the definition of the disorder.

Problems in the Behavioural Sciences

Theoretical approaches to obsessive-compulsive disorder

Problems in the Behavioural Sciences

Theoretical approaches to obsessive-compulsive disorder

Ian Jakes
Goldsmith's College, University of London

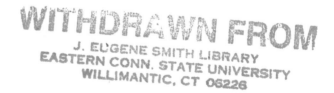
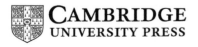

CAMBRIDGE
UNIVERSITY PRESS

Published by the Press Syndicate of the University of Cambridge
The Pitt Building, Trumpington Street, Cambridge CB2 1RP
40 West 20th Street, New York, NY 10011-4211, USA
10 Stamford Road, Oakleigh, Melbourne 3166, Australia

First published 1996

Printed in the United States of America

Library of Congress Cataloging-in-Publication Data
Jakes, Ian.
Theoretical approaches to obsessive-compulsive disorder / Ian Jakes.
p. 9 cm. – (Problems in the behavioural sciences: 14)
Includes biographical references.
ISBN 0-521-46058-1 (hc)
1. Obsessive-compulsive disorder. I. Title. II. Series.
RC533. J35   1996
616.85'227 – dc20   95-52163
                                                        CIP

A catalog record for this book is available from the British Library

ISBN 0-521-46058-1 Hardback

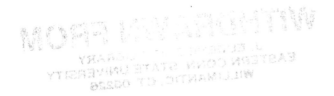

Ian Jakes was an exceptionally gifted young scientist and clinician who died tragically at the age of 34, shortly after the manuscript of this book had been delivered to the publishers. Ian's close colleague and mentor, Padmal de Silva, kindly undertook the task of steering the book through to the final printed version.

JEFFREY A. GRAY

Ian Jakes (1960–1995) studied psychology and philosophy at Cambridge University and then joined the Institute of Psychiatry, University of London, for postgraduate training in clinical psychology. After qualifying, he stayed on to carry out research into obsessive-compulsive disorder, leading to his Ph.D. At the time of his death resulting from acute leukaemia in April 1995, he was working both as a University lecturer and a clinical psychologist. This book represents some of the theoretical work done by Ian in the last years of his life. It provides an incisive and constructive critique of the major theoretical approaches to obsessive-compulsive disorder. Those interested in obsessive-compulsive disorder, whether from a theoretical, clinical or research perspective, will find this book invaluable.

PADMAL DE SILVA

Department of Psychology
Institute of Psychiatry
University of London

To my parents, Charles and Ruth Jakes

Contents

The best lack all conviction, while the worst
Are full of passionate intensity

W. B. Yeats
"The Second Coming"

Synopsis of *Theoretical approaches to obsessive-compulsive disorder*

This book discusses the diagnostic criteria for, and a variety of theoretical accounts of, obsessive-compulsive disorder (OCD).

The definition of OCD

It is suggested that the existing defining criteria for OCD are inadequate, that there is no single set of features that is both common and peculiar to all instances of the disorder, and that there is no single way in which OCD may be distinguished from phobic or delusional states; a number of different ways in which these distinctions between OCD and other states may be drawn are noted.

The approach to the definition of OCD that is defended here may, in suggesting that no single set of features is both common and peculiar to all instances of the disorder, be similar to the definition of schizophrenia that is offered by DSM-III-R – both definitions provide, that is, what DSM-III-R terms polythetic criteria.

It is not suggested that the subdivisions of OCD symptoms, of which the definition that is offered here is composed, are important from the point of view of such matters as the explanation or treatment of the disorder. It is too early to claim any such importance for these subdivisions, and indeed, it is argued that any differences among OCD patients in terms of the aetiology and/or treatment of their disorder may turn out to be unrelated to differences in the kinds of symptoms they report.

Behavioural/learning accounts of OCD

It is argued that most of those aspects of the behavioural/learning account of OCD that are considered here meet with substantial difficulties. This account is correct in suggesting that many obsessions and compulsions are provoked by environmental cues and that exposure to these cues causes many patients to experience discomfort. It is argued, however, that attempted explanations of the repetitiveness of some compulsions from a behavioural point of view are implausible and that behavioural/learning theorists may have exaggerated the importance of discomfort reduction to the maintenance of compulsive behaviour. Discomfort reduction is not necessary to explain the maintenance of such behaviour, and some brief remarks are offered as to how a common explanation might be provided for the maintenance of both discomfort-reducing and discomfort-increasing compulsions.

The behavioural/learning approach encounters difficulties in explaining both the selectivity of OCD's feared stimuli and the paradoxical failures of these stimuli to extinguish. It is argued that the incubation and preparedness hypotheses fail to meet these difficulties.

It is noted that the behavioural/learning account is not unique in providing an explanation of why exposure with response prevention should be effective with OCD; other accounts are able to provide alternative explanations. Accounts by behavioural theorists of those obsessions that are not provoked by environmental cues have helped to inspire a new approach to the treatment of such obsessions. The efficacy of this approach has as yet not been established, however, and it is argued that behavioural accounts, which stress the supposed similarities between these kinds of obsessions and phobic objects, fail to explain why such obsessions should occur. Doubts are also raised as to the value of an alternative theoretical approach in which obsessions are seen as a sign of unprocessed emotion. Some further work by behaviour therapists is noted in connection with Janet's account of OCD.

The cognitive-behavioural approach

It is argued that the cognitive-behavioural account provides no very compelling reason for supposing the appraisals it presents in the case of some instances of OCD (those involving blasphemous, sexual or aggressive obsessions) either to be the primary source of distress or to be the mechanism, in conjunction with neutralising behaviour, that converts normal obsessions of this kind into abnormal obsessions. The interesting connection between some aspects of the cognitive-behavioural account as applied to cases of this kind, and the observation that OCD patients are sometimes people of "tender conscience", is noted. A possible alternative explanation of OCD's occurring in such people is also briefly considered. In other cases of OCD, it is argued, the appraisals cited by the cognitive-behavioural account describe what needs to be explained, rather than provide an explanation. The cognitive-behavioural account, in making many of the same assumptions as the behavioural/learning approach, may also face some of the difficulties that approach encounters – for example, it may, in its present form, share the inability of the behavioural/learning approach to explain the repetitiveness of some compulsive behaviour.

Accounts of OCD based upon personality theories derived from the work of Pavlov

Accounts from the perspective of Pavlovian personality theories suggest that OCD patients should tend to be introverted, but evidence is presented that contradicts this claim. From the evidence quoted, introversion appears to be exhibited more by those OCD patients whose major difficulty is cleaning than it is by those whose major difficulty is checking. This, of course, leaves open the possibility that the neuroticism of OCD patients may play a role in producing their symptoms, as writers such as Eysenck, Claridge and Gray suggest, and indeed, it may even be (once again consistent with the views of Eysenck, Claridge and Gray) that in those OCD patients in whom both introversion and neuroticism occur, these two features combine to play a role in producing the symptoms observed. But even if all of this is accepted, it is clear that such temperamental characteristics as neuroticism and introversion cannot deliver a full account of the symptoms reported by OCD patients. Thus, these temperamental characteristics are supposed to be exhibited not only by patients suffering from OCD, but also by patients with other dysthymic disorders, and so these characteristics could not begin to explain why, for example, one patient develops neurotic depression or a phobia while another develops OCD. Similarly, there appears to be a wide gulf between the mere emotional reactivity that is supposed to characterise neurotic introverts, on the one hand, and, on the other, the bizarre preoccupations, repetitive behaviour and failures of memory that are reported by many OCD patients.

It is this gulf that Gray's account attempts to bridge, whereas Claridge tries both to do this and to explain – in terms of individual differences in attentional style – why some patients develop OCD rather than phobias or depression. Both of these accounts, it is argued, meet with difficulties. Gray's appears for a number of reasons not to provide a plausible explanation of the various OCD symptoms he discusses, including those that involve checking difficulties – the phenomena for which this account at first appears to provide an especially elegant explanation. It is noted that Claridge's account possesses a number of important strengths but relies too heavily on Reed's formulation of obsessional difficulties, thus encountering a number of the problems faced by that formulation.

What may be the most powerful argument considered in this discussion of personality theories derived from the work of Pavlov owes very little directly to those personality theories, this argument being that it may be possible to explain the contents of some OCD symptoms (particularly those involving, as Gray suggests, fears of dirt/contamination and/or cleaning behaviour) in terms of the evolutionary advantage that such fears and behaviour may be hypothesised to have bestowed. It is also noted, however, that the contents of various other OCD symptoms could not be explained in these terms. In those cases where evolutionary arguments do possess some force, it is suggested, once again consistent with Gray's and some of Claridge's remarks, that the most plausible mechanism through which such evolutionary pressures could exercise this influence may be that of innately acquired, rather than prepared, fears.

Janet on OCD

Janet included OCD, among other conditions, in the category he termed *psychasthenia*. Pitman praises the clinical astuteness of Janet's work and suggests that it is not so much Janet's theory of psychasthenia, but rather his observations and treatment suggestions concerning the disorder, that have stood the test of time. Janet's theory of psychological tension and his speculations as to a physiological tension corresponding to it, were, according to Pitman, an unsuccessful attempt to make sense of Janet's observations concerning psychasthenic patients. Some of these observations, however, such as those concerning the interpersonal difficulties encountered by these patients and the co-morbidity of the various symptoms they report, remain important contributions. In the light of Reed's interpretation, it needs to be added that opinions differ on how Janet's theory of psychasthenia is to be understood, but this turns out not to be a reason for questioning Pitman's lack of confidence in the theory – Reed's own account of OCD, which has much in common with his interpretation of Janet, meets with substantial difficulties. It is of interest that some of Pitman's suggestions as to the nature of OCD, made while outlining a cybernetic model of the disorder, have some similarities with Reed's account. It is also noted that the account of some symptom contents to which Janet was led by his theory of psychological tension may have been too readily rejected by writers such as Pitman. Something like Pitman's psychodynamic account, on the one hand, and Janet's account, on the other, may provide contrasting predictions as to the likely outcome of using assertion training with some (but not all) of the psychasthenic patients described by Janet. It is noted that some behaviour therapists have used this intervention with OCD patients (also see later).

Doubts have been raised regarding the extent to which Janet's treatment suggestions amount to the recommendation to use exposure with response prevention with OCD patients. Concerning Janet's clinical observations, doubts have also been raised as to the extent to which these would apply to all OCD patients.

Pitman's cybernetic model of OCD

In presenting a cybernetic model of OCD, Pitman discusses a number of interesting cases where symptoms involve indecisiveness, perfectionism and conflict. But, insofar as the cybernetic model makes substantive suggestions as to the explanation of OCD – in terms of a postulated internal comparator mechanism containing a fault that makes it more difficult to extinguish error signals – it encounters a number of difficulties, the most important of these being in making sense of the motivation of patients suffering from the disorder. Insofar as these difficulties are avoided – by supposing the internal comparator fault to produce error signals that are, in contrast, abnormally strong, or by presenting the cybernetic model within a "conflict/displacement" account – it appears that the cybernetic component of these accounts fails to make any substantive contribution to them. In its present form, therefore, it must be concluded that the model does not significantly advance our understanding of OCD.

A psychodynamic approach to OCD

Some psychodynamic theories of OCD are briefly outlined, and a case discussion presented by Malan is examined in some detail. Four features, it is argued, give this case discussion its psychodynamic character. These four features are the account's reference to unconscious mental processes, its formulation of the patient's concerns as having symbolic significance, its claim that the patient's difficulties may be understood as having occurred in order to serve some purpose for him, and its claim that insight into hidden feelings derived from childhood experience is of fundamental importance to therapeutic outcome. It is argued that, if there is anything of a psychodynamic character about the first of these features, this is merely a semantic matter. The other three features are all more substantial, but reasons are offered for thinking none of them to be important to the understanding of the case presented by Malan. The possible relevance of this case to the understanding of OCD in general is discussed.

There are links between some of Malan's remarks, and Freud's ideas concerning the anal-sadistic stage and OCD – in particular, the emphasis in Malan's account on the patient's supposed efforts to control his own anger, and Malan's relating this to the theme of the elimination of body products. Reasons for accepting an alternative account of the exaggerated importance of body products are offered.

One might, then, conclude that doubts are justified as to the psychodynamic aspects of Malan's account.

These points do certainly not imply that Malan's discussion fails in all respects to illuminate OCD. Some of Malan's remarks seem as if they may do so – in particular, his suggestions that unassertive behaviour may be important in understanding some cases of OCD and that encouraging constructive assertion may be a useful intervention for these cases.

Cognitive style/deficit approaches to OCD: Reed's account

Reed originally argued that obsessional disorders all stem from difficulties in the spontaneous structuring of experience, which in turn lead to compensatory over-structuring. Reed himself later pointed out that this hypothesis, as it stands, makes poor sense of some cases, especially those involving checking and rumination. He attempted to remedy this by supplementing his account with the concept of redintegration. It is suggested that this supplement is implausible. It is also argued that Reed's account makes poor sense of OCD symptoms in which doubts, indecision and ritualising do not play a major role or do not appear at all. Certain aspects of some of the OCD symptoms that do involve these characteristics, furthermore, are not explained by this account – in particular, the fact that, in many cases, certain themes tend to feature (that is, OCD's feared stimuli exhibit selectivity) and the fact that these difficulties sometimes involve just a few areas of the patient's life.

It is argued that Reed's hypothesis also fails to explain the motivation of OCD patients in carrying out their compulsive behaviour. A suggested revised version of Reed's thesis can explain why at least some OCD patients are highly motivated to behave as they do, but this thesis fails to account for various observations – once again, especially those that tend to be associated with checking difficulties. It is argued that a partial explanation of such difficulties from this perspective may be possible, however. This revised thesis is also argued to be poor at distinguishing OCD patients from other psychiatric groups, including phobic and deluded subjects.

The type of laboratory evidence Reed presents in favour of his thesis is argued to provide only weak support, while the clinical observations Reed cites to this same end are at best controversial. Laboratory evidence is introduced that is inconsistent with that cited by Reed. Objections are brought against Reed's comments as regards the use of behavioural and cognitive therapy and the use of assertiveness training with OCD.

It is also argued that Reed's account misrepresents the role of anxiety in OCD and carries implausible implications as to the relationship both between OCD and the obsessional personality/personality disorder and between OCD, on the one hand, and anxiety and depressive disorders, on the other.

A number of further comments are offered on Reed's discussion of external structuring; his interpretation of Janet; his account of the experience of compulsion; and his comments on the definition of OCD as well as on the definitions of the obsessional personality and personality disorder.

What of Reed's account may be salvaged from the foregoing discussion? The account appears to be most plausible when regarded as a partial explanation of some OCD difficulties – in particular, those where one observes the patient's having, in Reed's terms, problems structuring some task and tending to perform it in an overstructured manner. Among the best examples of cases of this kind appear to be some instances involving contamination fears and cleaning behaviour.

The revised thesis seems most likely to provide a full explanation in the case of those OCD symptoms where some unlikely outcome is feared by the patient, but where neither constant doubts about, nor endless repetitions of, compulsive behaviours are observed. Many cases involving cleaning difficulties correspond to this profile.

Both Reed's account and the revised thesis, therefore, seem to be most plausible in many cases of cleaning difficulties. It needs to be stressed, however, that the greater plausibility of these approaches as regards cleaning problems really amounts to no more than the absence of the objections that arise regarding the application of Reed's account and the revised thesis to other kinds of difficulties, such as checking behaviours and discrete obsessional thoughts, images and impulses. There are, that is, no positive grounds for accepting either of these approaches even in the case of cleaning problems, and it remains entirely possible, therefore, that the cognitive factors discussed by Reed will turn out to be entirely secondary phenomena in OCD, playing only a minor, or even no, role (when they appear at all) in producing the pathological thinking and behaviour that is observed.

Biological approaches to OCD

A variety of biological findings concerning OCD patients, and proposed animal models of these patients, are considered, along with a number of the psychological accounts of OCD that are offered by biological theorists. It is argued that these biological findings, if sound, would support the claims of some biological theorists that abnormalities in the basal ganglia, and perhaps also the frontal cortex, play some role in producing and maintaining OCD; these biological findings are not, however, subject to either detailed or comprehensive scrutiny here. Claims that the limbic system may also be involved in causing OCD (a claim also made by Pavlovian personality theorists) are also considered, and some possible difficulties for these claims are noted. As regards the psychological accounts that are considered, it is suggested that a conflict/displacement approach is perhaps the most plausible; nonbiological work that may support this approach is noted.

Concluding remarks

Can an example be provided, then, from among these various theoretical approaches to OCD, of some ideas concerning the disorder that are shared by a number of these approaches and that, while no doubt failing to provide a complete account of OCD, can be said to have made some progress in understanding the disorder? One example is considered. It has been pointed out in connection both with Janet's discussion of OCD and with Malan's psychodynamic approach, that a tendency to unassertiveness is observed in some OCD patients. These approaches suggest that a failure to act assertively and/or to express aggressive feelings may help precipitate the symptoms of some OCD patients and that these symptoms may, therefore, be alleviated by an intervention that successfully encourages these patients to behave more assertively and/or to express their aggressive feelings to a greater extent. Similar suggestions have been made by some behaviour therapists who use assertiveness training with OCD patients, and some aspects of the psychological accounts offered on the basis of biological research into the disorder also overlap to some extent with these suggestions. These ideas are critically discussed. An attempt is made to show that at least some of these suggestions are theoretically progressive – that is, that they offer explanations and predictions that cannot readily be supported by other accounts of OCD; this is followed by a few remarks as to whether or not these suggestions may also be regarded as empirically progressive – whether or not, that is, the explanations and predictions that are provided by these suggestions have been confirmed.

Acknowledgments, and provenance of *Theoretical approaches to obsessive-compulsive disorder*

My thanks are especially due to Dr Gerry Riley, Dr Philippa Garety, Professor Jeffrey Gray, my PhD examiners (Professor Ray Hodgson and Dr Derek Bolton), my PhD supervisors (Professor David Hemsley and Mr Padmal de Silva), Mr Andrew Clay, and Ms Roz Shafran.

Except for Chapter 7, this book is based on work included in my PhD thesis. Additions to, and alterations of, the material from my thesis have been carried out for Chapters 5 and 8.

Some of Chapter 1 has already been published as an article, "The definition of obsessive-compulsive disorder", by the *Journal of Mental Health* (1994) 3, pp. 287–99.

1   The natural history and definition of obsessive-compulsive disorder

1.1   Introduction and natural history

It is quite common for books on obsessive-compulsive disorder (OCD) to open by offering a brief definition of the disorder. Because the definition of OCD is to be treated here as a major issue in its own right, such an introduction is not possible. Instead, a few examples of symptoms reported by OCD patients are offered. A fuller picture of the symptoms reported by these patients will be provided by the discussion of the definition of the disorder later in this chapter. All the following examples are taken from de Silva (1988, pp. 196–7):

(a) thought plus... [mental] image [of the patient's having] knocked someone down with his car
(b) impulse...to shout obscenities during prayer or a church service
(c) [mental] image of corpses rotting away...
(d) repeated and extensive washing of hands to get rid of contamination by germs
(e) checking gas taps, door handles, and switches three times [whenever the patient]went past them
(f) imagining in sequence...photographs of members of [the patient's] family, his parents, pictures of Jesus Christ and the Virgin Mary, and then photographs of two other persons

Chapters 2 to 7 will review a variety of theoretical approaches to OCD. Although a diversity of work will be covered by this review, including behavioural, cognitive, psychodynamic, and biological approaches to the disorder, the review will not aim to be exhaustive. In particular, it will omit detailed consideration of such important elements as the interesting relationship between OCD and depression (Stengel, 1945; Lewis, 1934), and the phenomenological approach of Schneider (1925), whose classic work on personality disorders includes a discussion of obsessionals, termed by him insecure psychopaths. Chapter 8 will attempt to identify some converging lines of inquiry from the variety of theoretical approaches considered in the preceding chapters.

There are a number of summaries of the evidence available regarding the natural history of OCD (for example, Black, 1974; Rachman and Hodgson, 1980; Reed, 1985), and the findings reported in these summaries will not be repeated in detail here. OCD has traditionally been regarded as relatively rare, its prevalence among psychiatric out-patients estimated to be between 0.3% and 0.6% (de

Silva, 1988); its prevalence among in-patients is somewhat higher, but still under 5% (Black, 1974; Hare, Price, and Slater, 1972; Rachman and Hodgson, 1980). The prevalence of the disorder among the general population had been estimated to be about 0.05% (Rudin, 1953, quoted by Rasmussen and Eisen, 1990, p. 10), but the American Epidemiological Catchment Area (AECA) studies found a "strikingly high lifetime prevalence...ranging from 2% to 3%" (Bebbington 1990), with a six-month prevalence of 1.3–2.0% (Myers et al., 1984; Robins et al., 1984; Karno et al., 1988). These estimates suggest OCD to be "the fourth most common psychiatric disorder" after phobias, substance abuse, and major depressive disorder, its prevalence in the AECA studies being "twice that of schizophrenia or panic disorder" (Rasmussen and Eisen, 1990, p. 10).

Anthony et al. (1985), using psychiatrists rather than the lay interviewers recruited by the AECA surveys, suggest that these surveys may have overesti-mated the prevalence of OCD, but Rasmussen and Eisen cite still further epi-demiological work that is broadly consistent with those surveys. Bebbington (1990) examined the prevalence of OCD in a community in London, making a more detailed appraisal of the severity of the illness than that made by the AECA surveys. His lifetime prevalence estimate is also broadly in line with that of the AECA surveys, although Bebbington emphasises that most of the cases he iden-tified were relatively mild.

The AECA studies also found that males were affected by OCD in almost the same numbers as females, that the disorder was most commonly reported in the 25–40-year age group, that OCD was more common among whites than blacks, and that the disorder was equally common in all social classes. Rasmussen and Eisen (1990, p. 12) report the onset of OCD to be significantly earlier for men than it is for women; the average ages of onset are 17.5 years and 20.8 years respectively. Onset of OCD after the age of 45 has traditionally been held to be rare (Black, 1974; Rachman and Hodgson, 1980 – but see Eaton et al., 1989).

Some further details concerning the natural history of OCD, in particular, what is known about the relationship between OCD and the obsessional person-ality (and personality disorder), are offered in Sections 4.3.1 and 6.12.

De Silva (1988, p. 203) notes two factors (among others) that may, he suggests, "influenc[e] the aetiology" of OCD, these being precipitating stresses and genetic influences. Regarding the first of these factors, de Silva (1988) notes that in many cases no specific time of onset can be established. In those cases where such a time can be identified, however, general stresses like "overwork, sexual and martial problems...[and] the illness [or] death of a close relative" (de Silva, 1988, p. 203) are sometimes present, suggesting that in these cases such difficulties may have helped to precipitate the disorder. Reed (1985, p. 70) suggests that reports differ as to which of these kinds of stress are most common at the onset of OCD. It might be argued, of course, that such difficulties as overwork and sexual or marital problems, are themselves produced by the onset of OCD. But this position may be at least in part controverted by McKeon, Roa, and Mann's (1984) finding that OCD patients with anxious premorbid personalities tend to experience fewer life events prior to the onset of their disorder than do patients with lower premorbid trait anxiety; this perhaps indicates a precipitating role for such events, with highly anxious personalities requiring fewer precipitants before developing OCD.

Turning to the second of the factors cited by de Silva, one can argue that the evidence for a "specific genetic contribution to obsessional-compulsive disorder is inconclusive" (Rachman and Hodgson, 1980, p. 41), because the studies of relevance to this matter have failed to control for possible environmental influences. Thus, there is no adequate control for such influences in the two studies whose findings are quoted by de Silva (1988) as possibly supporting a genetic contribution to OCD: Carey and Gottesman (1981), who reported the concordance of OCD to be higher among monozygotic twins than among dizygotic twins; and Murray et al. (1981), who reported a high concordance of "obsessionality" – traits and symptoms – among a large sample of normal twins. Rasmussen and Eisen (1990, p. 13) also suggest that two recent family studies show convincingly that OCD is familial. Environmental influences might evidently be able to explain all of these findings, and, as explained by de Silva (1988, p. 204), crucial studies, such as of monozygotic twins who have been reared apart, are lacking. Rachman and Hodgson point out that "there is plausible support for the argument that there is an important genetic contribution to *general* emotional oversensitivity or neuroticism" and suggest that "the possibility of a general genetic contribution [to OCD], through the vehicle of an increased predisposition to anxiety, or to neuroses generally, cannot be excluded" (1980, p. 41, original emphasis; see Chapter 3 for accounts that emphasise the role of neuroticism in OCD).

1.2   OCD: existing suggestions for the diagnostic criteria

1.2.1   Introduction

What follows is a critique of a number of definitions of OCD that are currently on offer. The distinction between OCD and "normal" obsessions and compulsions (Rachman and de Silva, 1978) will not be examined, this distinction being determined only by the relatively vague judgement as to whether or not the disruption in a person's functioning caused by his or her obsessions and/or compulsions is sufficiently severe for the symptom to be judged of clinical severity. Although the diagnostic criteria examined in this section and Section 1.3 will be referred to as those for OCD, they are, therefore, equally relevant to the task of identifying, among subclinical experiences and behaviour, those that are "normal" obsessions and compulsions. There will also be in this section no discussion of the definition of the obsessive-compulsive personality (Pollack, 1979, 1987; Reed, 1985) although some comments on this topic are offered later (see Section 6.12).

1.2.2   The major authorities

Snaith (1981) remarks that ever since the time that Esquirol first described a case and Morel first used the term *obsession* (also see Black, 1974), OCD has been subject to frequent redefinition. Other writers disagree; Rachman and Hodgson (1980) suggest that, since the introduction of the concept of *obsessional neurosis*, its definition has "produced little controversy". Reed (1985) also takes this line and argues that all the major authorities in this area – Westphal, Janet, Freud, Jaspers, Schneider, Lewis, and so forth – agree on the definition of the disorder (see Reed, 1985, pp. 1–4, for quotes from these authorities). Reed suggests that the same definition is also put forward by DSM-III (Diagnostic and Statistical Manual of Mental Disorders, 3rd Edition; although see Section 1.2.4).

Thus, according to Reed, all of these sources suggest that for any thought, act, impulse, image, and so forth to be symptomatic of OCD, it must

(1) have a "subjectively *compulsive quality*" – the person must feel "*compelled*, pressed or driven" to think or act as he does,
(2) be recognised by the person as "*senseless* or absurd" – insight is retained into the morbidity of the thought or action – and
(3) be resisted by the person – he must fight not to think or act as he does

(quoted passages from Reed, 1985, p. 4, emphasis in original).

1.2.3   Lewis on the definition of OCD

Although Snaith appears rather to exaggerate the extent of disagreement regarding the diagnostic criteria for OCD, Reed overstates the extent of agreement (although see his 1985 discussion, pp. 5–6). Lewis (1936), for example, states that Schneider's definition is at once "precise and practicable" (p. 325) but goes on to deny, against Schneider, that senselessness is essential; he further suggests that resistance is both essential and omitted by Schneider's criteria.

Attention must be drawn to the sense in which Lewis uses the term resistance in the frequently quoted passage from his 1936 paper. He says "there should...be mention of the feeling that one must resist the obsession. This resistance is experienced as that of one's free will. The innumerable devices, rituals, and repetitions of the obsessional are secondary expressions of this immediate experience; they carry into effect the urge to ward off the painful and overwhelming obsession. The more overwhelming and painful the obsession, the more urgent and unsuccessful the devices to ward it off" (Lewis, 1936, p. 325). Thus, the "devices, rituals and repetitions" of these patients are part of their resistance, according to Lewis; he is not arguing that these behaviours themselves have to be resisted.

This is in sharp contrast to the criteria presented by Reed, which state that for such behaviours to be symptomatic of OCD they must be resisted. This use of *resistance* by Lewis is evidently confusing. Consider, for example, the ritual checking of a plug socket in response to the obsessional doubt that the plug has not been removed. Such checking does not resist, or "carry into effect the urge to ward off", this doubt. On the contrary, it is a failure to resist it or to ward it off.

Reed's criteria are not alone in misrepresenting Lewis on this point. For example, Stern and Cobb (1978), in their comments on Lewis's views, take issue with his diagnostic criteria because of the response of their sample of OCD patients to "probing questions [that] were asked to determine whether the patient struggled against an internal resistance, or conversely just gave in and carried out the ritual activity" (1978, p. 235). On Lewis's use of *resistance,* these questions would be incoherent.

1.2.4 The DSM-III-R criteria: the separate definitions of obsesssion *and* compulsion

The definitions of *obsession* and *compulsion* are given separately by DSM-III-R, as they are by DSM-III and by Rachman and Hodgson (1980), among other authorities. These sources restrict the former term to those OCD symptoms that are involuntary or "passive" (de Silva, 1988, p. 196), and the latter term to those that are voluntary or "active" (de Silva, 1988, p. 196). Compulsions are voluntary or active in that the patient can choose, albeit usually with difficulty, not to perform them; obsessions are involuntary or passive in that no such choice can be exercised by the patient regarding them. DSM-III, DSM-III-R, and Rachman and Hodgson also suggest a number of other additions to the criteria presented by Reed.

To illustrate the distinction between obsession and compulsion that is being drawn, a checker's thought that his door may be unlocked would be regarded as an obsession; his act of checking the door as a result of this thought would be regarded as a compulsion. Although DSM-III-R is not explicit on the point, its definition does not require compulsions to be overt behaviour. Thus, mental activity that is voluntary – for example, counting to oneself to avoid misfortune – is compulsive, according to DSM-III-R's definition. Compulsions may be, then, either overt (that is, behavioural) or covert (that is, mental), whereas obsessions are always covert (that is, mental), according to this definition (the same is true of the definition offered by DSM-III).

DSM-III defined obsessions as "recurrent, persistent ideas, thoughts, images, or impulses that are ego-dystonic, that is, they are not experienced as voluntarily produced, but rather as thoughts that invade consciousness and are experienced as senseless or repugnant. Attempts are made to ignore or suppress them" (p. 234). This passage is slightly modified in DSM-III-R, which states that obsessions need only be *initially* experienced as "intrusive and senseless" (p. 245). The DSM-III/III-R criteria add that a person must recognise his thoughts, impulses, and so on, to be the product of his own mind if these are to be symptomatic of OCD. Rachman and Hodgson (1980, p. 2) similarly suggest that the diagnostic criteria for obsessions are "intrusiveness, internal attribution, unwantedness and difficulty of control". A variation on this also used by these authors is that obsessions are "intrusive, unwanted thoughts, images or impulses which are unacceptable and/or unwanted". Rachman and Hodgson add that "internal resistance, and rejection of the idea...as alien and/or unrealistic [are] confirmatory indicators" of the idea in question being an obsession.

Turning now to the separate definition of compulsions offered by these sources, DSM-III-R defines these as "repetitive, purposeful, and intentional behaviours that are performed in response to an obsession, according to certain rules, or in a stereotyped fashion" (p. 245). It adds that such behaviour must be "performed with a sense of subjective compulsion that is coupled with a desire to resist the compulsion (at least initially)" and that "the person [must recognise] that his or her behaviour is excessive or unreasonable" (p. 245). DSM-III-R also requires that patients "do not derive pleasure from carrying out [a compulsion], although it provides a release of tension" (p. 245). (Lewis [1936, p. 326] similarly notes that the more the doing of an act is enjoyed, the less that act is like a compulsion.) Rachman and Hodgson (1980, p. 2) offer very similar criteria for the definition of compulsion.

This account of the concept of OCD is not dramatically altered by the definition offered in DSM-IV (1994). For example, this too suggests that obsessions "are persistent ideas, thoughts, impulses, or images that are experienced as intrusive and inappropriate and that cause marked anxiety or distress" (p. 418) and suggests that compulsions "are repetitive behaviours...or mental acts...the goal of which is to prevent or reduce anxiety or distress, not to provide pleasure or gratification" (p. 418). DSM-IV, like DSM-III-R, holds that "by definition, adults with Obsessive-Compulsive Disorder have at some point recognised that the obsessions or compulsions are excessive and unreasonable" (p. 418). DSM-IV includes a "specifier" – "With Poor Insight" – in its definition of OCD, to be applied when a current episode of the disorder is mainly unaccompanied by the patient's recognition of the excessive or unreasonable nature of his or her symptoms; DSM-IV suggests (p. 421) that this specifier "may be useful in those situations that are on the boundary between obsession and delusion". (DSM-IV thus suggests, with Reed [see Chapter 6] that insight occurs on a continuum.) The following discussion will be concerned with the details of the DSM-III-R definition of OCD; most of the same points could also be made regarding DSM-IV's account.

The three criteria presented by Reed – along with the distinction between obsessions and compulsions (and the other additions) suggested by the DSM criteria and by Rachman and Hodgson's definition – will be referred to as the "standard" diagnostic criteria in what follows. (See Walker,1973, and Snaith, 1981, for interesting alternative approaches to the definition of OCD.)

1.2.5 *The ordinary uses of* obsession *and* compulsion

It is worth noting in passing that the distinction made between the uses of the terms *obsession* and *compulsion* by the DSM-III-R criteria and Rachman and

Hodgson (1980) is stipulative, the employment of *obsession* and *compulsion* in ordinary (nonpsychiatric) discourse presenting no such distinction. Purposeful activity by which a person is preoccupied to an unusual degree (for example, stamp collecting or jogging) may be described as that person's obsession, whereas strong urges (for example, to drink or smoke) may be described as compulsions, despite their not being in themselves purposeful or intentional behaviour.

Other distinctions are also apparent among the ordinary uses of *obsession, compulsion,* and related locutions such as "being obsessed by", or "feeling compelled to do", something. One may be described as "feeling compelled" to do anything one is strongly inclined to do – for example, acting on a moral principle, smoking a cigarette, reading something of great interest. The activity in question might be unusual irrational, or unwanted, but equally it might not. To say that somebody "feels compelled" to do something is neutral as to these points. This is not true as regards somebody's "having an obsession with", or "being obsessed by", some thought or activity. One would not say this of a person's commitment to a moral principle, for example, if one shared this commitment with this person. The same appears to be true of somebody's "having a compulsion" to do, or "being compulsive about" doing, something. These also imply something unwanted or irrational about the desire or behaviour in question.

1.2.6 Evaluation of the standard defining criteria

1.2.6.1 The DSM criteria: stipulation versus description

To begin with a few remarks specifically concerning the DSM-III-R diagnostic criteria, it might be suggested that the definition offered by this source stipulates rather than describes the diagnostic criteria for OCD, in contrast to those suggested by the other sources cited. This is the point of a manual such as DSM-III-R, it might be argued – the manual is intended to instruct clinicians, not to give an account of what they do. On this view, the question of the validity of the DSM criteria would clearly not arise (where the "validity" of a given set of criteria is understood to mean how good a description of an existing concept these criteria provide). In what follows it will be assumed that the question of the validity of the DSM criteria does arise. This is to assume that if the decisions of experienced diagnosticians agree with one another but do not meet the DSM criteria, this is bad news for these criteria, not the diagnosticians. This assumption, then, gives the DSM criteria the descriptive status shared by all the other sources mentioned previously.

The exception to this "descriptive status" is the distinction the DSM criteria draw between obsession and compulsion, which is, as has already been pointed out, stipulative. This distinction is useful in highlighting an important distinction among the symptoms of OCD and is, on these grounds, justified. This distinction will be adopted in the following discussion, and all criticisms of the DSM criteria should be understood as not applying to it.

In what follows, it will be argued that the decisions of experienced diagnosticians do indeed not square with the standard diagnostic criteria, which have been outlined previously. It is important to be clear that this is not to claim that most diagnosticians, if asked, would agree that these criteria do not give a good account of their decisions. Quite probably they would say that these criteria do agree with their diagnostic practice, or they would at least regard them as giving an account of this practice that is sufficiently accurate to be useful for ordinary purposes. But it will be argued in what follows that, if one examines which patients are and are not actually classified as suffering from OCD, it can be seen that this classification is far more subtle and complex than the standard criteria allow, to the extent that these criteria cannot be regarded as providing even a rough approximation of the concept. It is, of course, neither a paradox nor a surprise that at least some diagnosticians will not themselves be aware that this is so. The ability to use a concept correctly does not imply the possession of an explicit account of that use.

The standard defining criteria will be evaluated first as regards obsessions and then as regards compulsions. This will, of course, mean two separate evaluations of the three criteria presented in Reed's review of the major authorities who do not distinguish between obsessions and compulsions.

1.2.6.2 Obsessions

If the very similar definitions of obsession suggested by DSM-III-R and Rachman and Hodgson (1980) are put together with the three criteria from Reed's discussion, the list of diagnostic features provided is as follows:

(a) a "subjectively compulsive" quality
(b) intrusiveness
(c) unwantedness or unacceptability
(d) difficulty in being controlled
(e) repetitiveness
(f) persistence
(g) internal attribution, or recognition as the product of one's own mind
(h) senselessness: recognised as senseless, or rejected as unrealistic or alien
(i) resistance: resisted, or attempts made to ignore or suppress

These nine criteria, it is to be argued, fail to provide the sufficient conditions for a definition of obsession. Some of them, it will be further argued, are not exhibited by every instance of OCD and are in this sense also not necessary for the diagnosis.

Consider first the claim that these features do not provide the sufficient conditions for this definition. These features do not distinguish obsessions from, for example, many phobic experiences. Take the example of an agoraphobic approaching a crowded shop. He may well experience such thoughts as "I may lose control and panic", "I may be sick", "I may go mad", "I may faint," and so forth. He may also experience images that concern these same themes. It is not being claimed – nor is it necessary for the present argument to claim – that these phobic thoughts and images will always meet all of the criteria (a)–(i). All that needs to be shown, and what is indeed being suggested, is that such experiences will sometimes do so while still being recognisably part of a person's phobic difficulties. Thus, the patient's phobic thoughts that he may, for example, panic and lose control will – working down the list from (a) to (i) – frequently be such that in this situation he feels compelled to think them while finding them intrusive, unwanted or unacceptable, difficult to control, repetitive and persistent. He will always recognise them as the product of his own mind and will at least sometimes also recognise them as senseless and resist them.

Going beyond this particular example, it is difficult to think of anyone's experiencing any significant degree of distress – be it anxiety, worry, anger, depression or whatever – without that person's thoughts at least frequently possessing features (a)–(f). The person's being nonpsychotic arguably guarantees that his thinking will possess feature (g) (also see Section 1.3.10), and features (h) and (i) are merely different ways in which a person may struggle with what he is thinking. Yet, whatever else we may mean by calling some aspect of a person's experience an obsession, it is clear that we must mean by this something more specific than that he has some nonpsychotic distress with which he is struggling. It may be concluded, therefore, that the criteria considered at the beginning of this section must be rejected as not providing the sufficient conditions for a definition of obsession.

What, then, of the claim that some of these features are not exhibited by every instance of OCD and are thus not necessary? A number of authors – for example, Stern and Cobb (1978), Walker (1973), and Jakes (1992, Chapter 2) – report a proportion of patients whose symptoms lack features (h): senselessness, and (i): resistance, and yet who have been classified by senior diagnosticians as suffering from OCD. Against such findings it might be pointed out that DSM-III-R qualifies the necessity for senselessness and resistance, claiming that these need be present only initially. Yet this claim seems to be made in the absence of any evidence that subjects who do not report senselessness and resistance would in all cases have once done so and would otherwise not have received the diagnosis of OCD. The same objection may be used against Reed's related reply (1985, pp. 5–7) that insight and resistance are both a matter of degree and may vary from time to time.

Consider now feature (e): repetitiveness. To be told that, for example, a mother's impulse to harm her child lacks this feature does not enable one to conclude that this impulse is not an obsession. It seems that such impulses might indeed occur only once on any particular occasion and that one would not, by virtue of this alone, wish to withhold a diagnosis of OCD.

1.2.6.3 Compulsions

Turning now to compulsions – that is, those OCD symptoms that are voluntary behaviour – the three standard criteria from Reed's discussion once again fail to provide the necessary and sufficient conditions for a definition. Thus, these criteria cannot be *sufficient* because, for example, many patients will report, as part of a phobic difficulty, that they feel *compelled* to escape from their feared objects while at least sometimes trying to resist this feeling and also at least sometimes regarding it as *senseless*. Resistance and senselessness are also not necessary features of compulsions – the work of Stern and Cobb (1978), Walker (1973), and Jakes (1992, Chapter 2) quoted previously is again relevant here. DSM-III-R qualifies the necessity for these features and suggests that compulsions must at least be resisted initially, but, as with the similar claim made regarding obsession, this suggestion is unsubstantiated.

What of some of the additional features for the definition of compulsion, which are suggested by DSM-III-R to be necessary – that compulsions must be performed in response to an obsession, according to certain rules or in a stereotyped fashion? Do these three features take us any closer to a satisfactory definition of compulsion? It seems not. Although compulsions certainly may be performed according to certain rules or in a stereotyped fashion, both of these features appear to be absent in many patients. Indeed, the DSM-III-R definition may itself be consistent with this observation in that this definition seems to be a disjunction, rather than a combination, of these three features that is being put forward as necessary for a diagnosis of OCD.

To be successful, therefore, the DSM-III-R definition requires the third feature – that compulsions are carried out in response to obsessions – to be exhibited by all of those compulsions that fail to exhibit the other two features. But this third feature is uninformative, given that the urge to perform a compulsion is itself an obsession. One is not told, that is, how to distinguish urges to perform compulsive actions from urges to perform other kinds of behaviour. This distinction presupposes a definition of obsession that has not as yet been provided by either DSM-III-R or the other sources quoted earlier.

1.2.7 Implications of these criticisms

Raising these doubts as to the defining criteria for OCD is no mere semantic exercise. Substantial questions may be raised in both research and therapy by how the phenomena that are being investigated and treated are defined. In order to illustrate this claim, consider a contribution to the literature on OCD by Rachman and Parkinson (1981). It seems that this contribution makes some important errors and that it does so because of the definition of OCD with which its authors are working. This definition is the one suggested by Rachman and Hodgson (1980), which was quoted among the standard diagnostic criteria. Error results in the case of Rachman and Parkinson's (1981) work from their treating these criteria as providing the sufficient conditions for a diagnosis of the disorder; quite different problems may arise from regarding these criteria as necessary (see Section 6.7).

Rachman and Parkinson (1981) present the following anxious thoughts (among others), all of which were reported by mothers concerning their children who were at the time in hospital for surgery: "Ever since I knew she was booked in I have been thinking what might go wrong with the anaesthetic and surgery." (The same mother is reported as having a "repetitive image" in which "I have seen her lying there like a vegetable and not coming round from the operation".) "I have this repeated image of K. on a trolley, and they put him in a bed and then I see the blood everywhere. I try hard to clear it from my mind. The image frightens the life out of me." "It's been on my mind the whole time. I haven't been able to stop myself thinking about him and his operation." "I was thinking about it all the time. I was constantly going through in my mind how I would explain things to him. I keep seeing him in his gown, asleep, being taken down the theatre. I've seen him go down in my mind." "I keep hearing him and seeing him in hospital, crying." (All quotes from Rachman and Parkinson, 1981, p. 115 and p. 117.)

It should be noted that these thoughts would likely not meet one of the criteria specified by the standard definitions of OCD, that of senselessness (P. de Silva, personal communication, 1989). The women in Rachman and Parkinson's study, that is, would presumably regard their thoughts of their sick children as entirely reasonable material to have on their minds. Otherwise, however, these thoughts and images would at least very often satisfy the remaining criteria suggested by the standard definitions of OCD. Thus, referring back to the list of defining criteria for obsession presented earlier, these thoughts would usually have a "subjectively compulsive" quality and be experienced as intrusive, unwanted or unacceptable, repetitive and persistent. These thoughts would similarly be difficult to control, be recognised by these women as the products of their own minds, and attempts would, finally, also be made by these women to resist (that is, to ignore or suppress) these thoughts, as indeed was explicitly stated in some of the quotes.

It is *because* the thoughts reported by these women do largely satisfy the standard definitions of OCD that these authors are led to regard them as a *normal analogue* of OCD – to regard them, in other words, as "normal obsessions" (Rachman and de Silva, 1978). Thus, Rachman and Parkinson say as regards these thoughts that "the present study is designed to extend our comprehension of obsessions along what might be described as a normal dimension" (Rachman and Parkinson, 1981, p. 111).

Having taken up this position, Rachman and Parkinson then attempt to use the close study of the thoughts and images experienced by these women to shed light on clinical obsessions. For example, they argue that the absence of depressed mood as a precipitant of these thoughts is evidence that this mood state may have had its importance as a precipitant of clinical obsessions overstated.

Is it not plausible, however, to argue that these thoughts and images are not obsessions and are not even similar to obsessions in many respects, contrary to the position of Rachman and Parkinson? These women are clearly anxious about their children, but nothing that has been said so far suggests that there is anything obsessional about this anxiety at all. In particular, and with the earlier criticisms of the standard definitions in mind, this is not suggested by the fact that these thoughts are experienced as repetitive and unwanted and so forth. It is not possible to infer anything about obsessions (clinical or otherwise) from the nature of these thoughts – or at least no such inference is possible without raising the question of whether or not nonobsessional anxiety and obsessions differ such that the inference is misleading. These women's thoughts and images are no more similar to obsessions than they are to many nonobsessional phenomena. Indeed, it seems likely that there is a greater similarity between these thoughts and images, on the one hand, and some nonobsessional phenomena (for example, generalized anxiety states, panic attacks, etc.), on the other, than there is between these thoughts and images, and obsessions (also see Section 1.3).

1.3   A different approach to the definition of OCD

1.3.1 Introduction: the approach to be adopted

In trying to argue in the previous section that the characteristics of senselessness and resistance are not exhibited by all OCD symptoms, the approach was adopted of referring to empirical work, which shows that some patients who have been classified by senior diagnosticians as having OCD do not report these characteristics as regards their symptoms. A different approach will be adopted to support the analysis of the concept of obsessive-compulsive disorder that is to follow. This analysis presupposes that it is possible to recognise, while having as yet no account of the diagnostic criteria for OCD, what are and what are not instances of the disorder. Thus, it is suggested that in this respect, the concept of obsessive-compulsive disorder is the same as such concepts as, for example, illness or intention – that is, one may recognise, for example, that a person with influenza is ill or that a given item of a person's behaviour is intentional under certain descriptions, without being able to state what it is for something to be an illness or for behaviour to be intentional. The ability to recognise illnesses and intentional behaviour usually rests on the possession of a tacit understanding of these concepts. What users of these terms possess, that is, are implicit criteria for the application of the terms *illness* and *intentional behaviour,* criteria that analyses of these concepts would endeavour to make explicit. This would be done by attempting to identify those features that are necessary for instances of illness and intentional behaviour to be recognised as such. To take an example, one might test, with real or imagined cases, whether we should still be able, using our tacit understanding of the concept of illness, to recognise influenza as an instance of this concept were it not to involve suffering and/or impairment of a person's functioning. In this way, it would be possible to establish whether or not suffering and impairment of functioning are among the implicit criteria we possess for the use of the term *illness.* The same approach will be adopted here for the analysis of the concept of obsessive-compulsive disorder, with our implicit understanding of this concept being similarly used in tests of real or imagined cases to make that understanding explicit.

A source of potential difficulty for this approach is that one is required, in adopting it, to assume that there will be a general agreement in the judgments of different diagnosticians as to what are, and what are not, instances of OCD. If a sufficient degree of disagreement were found to exist among diagnosticians, then the whole approach of appealing to the implicit criteria that are supposed to be in use would collapse, and it would have to be concluded that there is no established concept of obsessive-compulsive disorder at all. Until any such evidence of radical disagreement is found, however, one is entitled to proceed with appeals to implicit criteria on the tentative assumption that such evidence will not be forthcoming. It is worth noting in passing that this approach of appealing to implicit criteria has also been used earlier in this chapter without having been explicitly introduced there as such. For example, such an appeal was made in arguing that much thinking and behaviour that can be recognised as phobic meet (and thus call into question) the standard defining criteria for OCD.

1.3.2   No unitary criteria for OCD

What, then, are the defining criteria for OCD? The best response to this question is probably a refusal to answer it in that form. Philosophical work, most notably that of Wittgenstein (1953), rejects the assumption that there have to be common and peculiar characteristics shared by all the phenomena picked out by any given term. This assumption *is* made by the standard definitions of the concept of OCD considered earlier, and the present discussion intends to show that this assumption is indeed mistaken in this case. Thus, the central claim of this discussion will be that *features that are not common to all OCD symptoms will often play a part in determining that some symptoms are of that character.*

1.3.3   The limits of the present account of the definition of OCD

It is not intended that the discussion that follows should provide an exhaustive account of all of the features that have a part to play in defining thinking and behaviour as OCD; this discussion will instead focus mainly on the distinction between OCD and phobias, although a few remarks will also be made about the distinction between OCD and delusions. One should also note that there may be some OCD symptoms that do not possess any of the features to be outlined here; the following account of the distinction between OCD and phobias may not, therefore, be exhaustive.

Although the following discussion will not deal with the distinction between OCD and many nonphobic disorders, it is worth remarking that an examination will be included of the distinction between OCD and some anxiety symptoms that, in some cases, would probably be regarded as nonphobic. Examples of non-OCD symptoms of this kind that will be discussed are such fears as whether or not a close relative has come to harm and whether or not one is about to have a heart attack. (It is of course not being claimed that such symptoms should not be diagnosed as OCD by virtue of their involving such themes.) Fears such as whether or not one is about to have a heart attack or whether or not a relative has come to harm will for the sake of simplicity be referred to as "phobic" in what follows.

1.3.4 The distinction between phobias and OCD

1.3.4.1 Introduction

A number of features that play a part in distinguishing OCD from phobic states will be presented. To reiterate the central claim made in Section 1.3.2: for each of these features, it will be argued that (1) its presence is crucial to the distinction between phobic states and those instances of OCD that exhibit the feature in question, and (2) there are other instances of OCD symptoms that do not exhibit this feature at all.

Two points are worth stressing at the outset of this discussion. First, for the purposes of the present argument, it will only need to be suggested for each of the features that its presence is part of the reason for characterising as OCD those symptoms exhibiting the feature. A series of examples of OCD symptoms will be presented; it will be pointed out that each symptom exhibits a given feature that, it will be claimed, distinguishes it from phobic symptoms. But this is not to claim that the OCD symptom may be characterised as such by virtue of its exhibiting the feature in question alone. Attention is only being drawn to the feature that distinguishes that OCD symptom from phobic states. It may well be that other nonphobic emotions or behaviour can also be distinguished from phobias in the same way, without their being considered symptomatic of OCD. Distinguishing such nonphobic phenomena from OCD would clearly have to be based on other grounds. But it is not necessary, for the purposes of a discussion concerned only with the distinction between phobias and OCD, to explore what these other grounds will be. (There will nonetheless be reason for making just a few remarks concerning this question toward the end of the discussion.)

Secondly, it is not being suggested that phobic patients never report any thinking or behaviour that exhibits the characteristics to be discussed here. The claim is rather that, insofar as such thinking and behaviour are reported, the patient is having experiences, or is behaving in ways, that are not phobic in nature. A phobic diagnosis will be inadequate only if such experiences or behaviour are a sufficiently important source of distress for the patient.

1.3.4.2 Characteristic (i): symptoms that concern the exercise of one's own will

OCD symptoms may involve the sufferer's fearing that he may knife somebody, utter some obscenity, or do some other unacceptable thing. Sometimes an OCD patient will alternatively report fears as to terrible things that he thinks he may have already done.

Phobic symptoms may also involve, as these OCD symptoms do, a fear of unacceptable things one may do – an agoraphobic may report as part of her phobic state a fear that she will be sick, faint, panic, and so forth. But this is not to fear one's own future or past *intentional* action, as in the present examples of OCD symptoms. It seems that such a fear of one's own intentional behaviour is by definition not phobic, and this feature is consequently sufficient to distinguish those OCD symptoms that exhibit it from phobic states.

Rather than fearing what they might do or might have done, some OCD patients experience *impulses* to perform unacceptable actions. One can feel sure that such experiences are not phobic in character – there are, that is to say, by definition no phobic impulses of this kind.

1.3.4.3 Characteristic (ii): "covert object" of fear or discomfort

As noted in Section 1.2.6.2, phobics will frequently experience intrusive, repetitive, and unwanted thoughts and images of a distressing nature; for example, an agoraphobic approaching a crowded shop may experience thoughts of how she might be sick or faint in the shop, images of these things happening, and so on. How might such a patient's thoughts and images of what she thinks is going to happen to her be distinguished from such obsessions as the following?

(a) images of horribly mutilated dead bodies
(b) blasphemous thoughts
(c) unacceptable insults concerning, for example, the appearance or conduct of the patient's partner or close relatives
(d) number sequences and nonsense phrases that continually run through the patient's mind

The crucial difference between such experiences as these and phobic thinking seems to be that the latter refers to objective states of affairs that the patient fears she will have to encounter, and/or things that she fears may happen – often her fear will concern situations she knows she will have to encounter very soon, as in the foregoing example of the agoraphobic. To take some further examples, the phobic patient may think of, or picture, the spider that she knows she is going to have to confront, or imagine the heart attack that she thinks she is about to sustain, or the humiliation she thinks she is about to suffer in some social situation.

OCD thinking of the kind being considered in the present section is not like this – the distress it involves is not the result of its referring to possible or actual situations that the patient thinks might or will occur; the patient is distressed by the content of her thinking without its referring to possible or actual situations at all. In this sense, then, the patient's fear or discomfort may be said to have a "covert object", as suggested in the section title.

Thus, in the case of examples (b), (c) and (d), and in contrast to the examples of phobic thinking just considered, it is not the truth or possible truth of what has been thought that distresses the patient. Indeed, it is not even logically possible for number sequences and nonsense phrases to be true or false, and the same applies to many blasphemies and insults, too – for example, a patient to be discussed later had insulting, blasphemous thoughts consisting only of swear words addressed to Jesus Christ.

The distress in examples (b) and (c) seems rather to be a matter of the patient's regarding these thoughts as unacceptable (also see Section 2.8). Furthermore, if such thoughts occur frequently, the sheer frustration and the worry of having such unwanted matter constantly on her mind also seem likely to contribute to the patient's distress, and in the case of example (d), this seems likely to be the heart of the problem.

Example (a) is somewhat different, but even here the patient is not experiencing what phobic patients sometimes experience – such as an image of a close relative dead at home and, at the same time, intense anxiety that the relative has indeed died. The images experienced in example (a) are unaccompanied by such anxieties as this and distress the patient solely by virtue of their horrifying contents – they are not taken by the patient to represent any situation she thinks will or may come about. As with examples (b), (c) and (d), therefore, the distress involved does not have to do with the question of whether or not something will happen or will have to be confronted.

A phenomenon that may seem to be closely related to these examples is exhibited by those OCD patients who respond to their feared situations – in contrast to many phobics – by performing some *covert* activity, such as counting to themselves, rather than by carrying out some overt behaviour, such as escaping from the feared situation. But some phobics may also try to deal with their fears by taking covert action – for example, telling themselves that there is nothing of which they should be scared. What seems to secure an OCD diagnosis, as opposed to a phobic diagnosis, for some covert behaviour is thus not its being covert as such, but rather its being prompted by superstitious thinking as to what effect the covert action in question will have – for example, thinking that a feared situation may be rendered safe by the performance of the covert action. Rather than being included in the present section, therefore, such instances of OCD have to be included in the section that follows.

1.3.4.4 Characteristic (iii): superstitious and bizarre thinking

Some OCD patients report anxieties about outcomes that strike one not merely as rather unlikely but *bizarrely* unlikely; for example, removing small stones from pathways for fear that others will trip on them and come to serious harm, or carefully positioning books on shelves in case they should fall and badly hurt someone.

It is not, of course, being denied that phobics do sometimes fear unlikely outcomes; for example, heart attacks and strokes may be feared by phobic subjects who have every reason for believing themselves to be perfectly healthy in physical terms. What is being claimed is that by definition one does not encounter among phobic states the bizarre degree of unlikelihood seen in these OCD symptoms. This distinction is probably not a categorical matter, and this would render the difference between phobic states and those OCD symptoms that are to be distinguished from them in this way a matter of degree rather than kind.

Some justification should briefly be provided here for this claim that fears of having heart attacks or strokes do not involve the same degree of irrationality as do fears of people's coming to great harm as a result of tripping on tiny stones or having books fall on them from ordinary household shelves. This is shown to be so by its being common to know of others who have suffered the kinds of misfortune that preoccupy the phobic patients in these examples; the same clearly does not hold true for the examples of OCD preoccupations considered under the present heading. Nonetheless, there may undeniably be difficulties in the reliable assessment of how bizarre any given thought is (Kendler, Glazer, and Morgenstern 1983), and it must be conceded that, to the extent that this is so, any distinction that depends upon such assessment may be difficult to judge satisfactorily.

It may be easier to judge other cases in this category that involve not merely a greater degree of irrationality on the part of the OCD patient, but rather his behaving in an *entirely superstitious* manner; for example, positioning objects in a certain way in order to avoid bad luck or – to reintroduce the covert behaviour example referred to in Section 1.3.4.3 – counting to oneself to neutralise some perceived threat. (These actions are superstitious in being performed to bring about outcomes that it is impossible for such actions to bring about.) Phobic avoidance and escape by definition do not involve superstitious thinking. The patient may certainly entertain irrational ideas as to the outcome of his behaviour, such as thinking that he will avoid a heart attack by escaping from a crowded shop. Although irrational, such behaviour plainly falls short of being superstitious.

1.3.4.5 Characteristic (iv): repetitive behaviour

Some OCD patients carry out repetitive checks of, for example, plug sockets and light switches, doing so because they are unable to convince themselves either that they have carried out their earlier checks properly or that they have carried out these checks at all. Similarly, objects may be cleaned over and over again. Although phobics certainly do sometimes experience repetitive *thoughts*, as has been argued in Section 1.2.6.2, repetitive action of the kind being considered here is by definition not phobic in nature.

1.3.4.6 Characteristic (v): arrangement of objects

Some OCD patients report themselves to be unable to feel comfortable unless things in their environment are arranged in a set way – for example, unless all objects of a given kind are lined up, or all books and pieces of paper placed so that they are parallel to the edges of the tables on which they have been placed. Sometimes superstitious thinking may accompany such practices, in which case the behaviour would be classified under category (iii) (see Section 1.3.4.4). But some patients do not seem to arrange things for superstitious reasons – some report simply not being able to stand things being arranged in any other fashion.

Such discomfort is, by definition, not phobic. Phobic patients fear types of situations – for example, crowded shops or social interaction. But these situations are never identified by the exact arrangement of objects in them. Similarly, phobics may often fear objects or animals, but it is once again always the mere presence of the objects or animals, not their arrangement or exact position, that troubles these patients.

1.3.5   The independence of characteristics (i)–(v)

The central claim of the present argument does not require only that these various features do distinguish OCD symptoms from phobic states. It also requires that these features are independent of one another and are thus entirely different ways in which OCD symptoms are distinguished from phobic states. It is clear this is the case. Some of these features may of course sometimes occur together and be parts of the same symptom – for example, a patient may perform a superstitious ritual as a result of experiencing an impulse. But there is absolutely no necessity for these various features to occur together. It follows that the feature on the basis of which one case of OCD may be distinguished from phobic difficulties need not be exhibited at all by another case of OCD (and thus obviously plays no part in distinguishing that case from phobic difficulties). It may be concluded that the central claim of the present discussion (see Section 1.3.2) has been established – features that are not common to all OCD symptoms play a part in determining, in many cases, that a given symptom is OCD in character.

Indeed, it seems to be logically impossible for some of the features that have just been considered to form parts of the same symptom. The concerns of a patient whose symptoms exhibit characteristic (ii), for example, by definition do not involve his worrying whether or not some event has taken place or will take place. This means that a symptom that exhibits characteristic (ii) cannot also be a doubt that he has performed some terrible act or a fear that he may, or is about to, do so. His symptom can thus not exhibit characteristic (i).

1.3.6   Connecting themes between characteristics (i)–(v)

There is, then, no single feature or collection of features shared by all OCD phenomena by which they may all be distinguished from phobic states. This is not to deny, however, that there are themes that are shared by the various features discussed previously. Those symptoms that are included under categories (iii)–(v), for example, may all be said to be examples of various kinds of ritual.

The concept of ritual seems to be much like that of OCD, with those features that are crucial to the characterisation of some behaviour as ritualised not being exhibited at all by other examples of ritual behaviour.

Another characteristic is shared by many of the different kinds of OCD symptoms that have been presented, and this can be best introduced by first noting that all phobias may be satisfactorily described as fears of, or discomfort about, some external object or situation. (The term *external* is being used here as it was in the discussion of category [ii]. The bodily states that trouble some phobic patients are thus external in that they are not mental events.) In the case of many OCD symptoms, by contrast, this description is unsatisfactory – it omits, in various ways, some crucial aspect of such symptoms. This, then, is another link between many OCD symptoms – they cannot be satisfactorily described as fears of, or discomfort about, some external object or situation. The most obvious examples of OCD symptoms that cannot be so described are those that exhibit characteristic (ii) and thus, by definition, do not involve external objects or situations at all. Some symptoms exhibiting characteristic (i) are somewhat less obvious examples, in that they clearly do involve – in contrast to symptoms possessing characteristic (ii) – external situations (those that involve being with the person concerning whom the patient experiences his impulses or doubts about doing harm). But it is surely unsatisfactory simply to describe the patient as having a fear of the presence of the person concerned, because this suggests that there is something about that person the patient fears. The problem is, rather, a fear the patient has concerning himself and, in particular, how he will behave (or may have behaved).

Some of the symptoms that exhibit characteristic (iii) involve superstitious thinking – for example, positioning objects in a certain way in order to avoid bad luck. One might certainly say of a patient who exhibited such a symptom that he has a fear of objects not being positioned in a certain way, but this description once again omits the very heart of the symptom – the patient's magical thinking concerning the consequences of his arranging these objects in the manner he does.

Similarly, it is unsatisfactory to describe much of the repetitive checking that exhibits characteristic (iv) as a fear of, or discomfort about, leaving (or the possible consequences of leaving) light switches on, plugs in sockets, doors unlocked, and so forth. This description once again omits the central feature of the symptom – the repeated attempts of the patient to convince himself that light switches are off, doors locked, and so on. Repetitive checking of this kind implies some further difficulty other than fear or discomfort concerning the task in question; a difficulty in registering or remembering one's own behaviour is implied (see Section 2.5).

By contrast, three remaining examples of OCD symptoms can indeed be satisfactorily described as fears of, or discomfort about, external objects or situations. Thus, consider those symptoms exhibiting characteristic (iii), which involve concerns about bizarrely unlikely outcomes – concerns, as mentioned in earlier examples, such as whether or not people will come to serious harm through tripping on small stones or having books fall on them from household shelves. These kinds of symptom may be described perfectly accurately as a fear of, or discomfort about, these things' happening. This description does not leave out any crucial aspect of the symptom. The same applies to symptoms exhibiting characteristic (v), which can be satisfactorily described as fears of, or discomfort about, for example, all objects of a given kind being lined up, or all books and pieces of paper being placed so that they are parallel to the edges of tables. It may also be possible to argue the same point as regards at least some of the cleaning that exhibits characteristic (iv) (see Section 2.5), in contrast to the repetitive checking of plug sockets or light switches.

All three of these kinds of OCD symptoms, then (that is, those exhibiting characteristics [iii] and [v], and at least some of the cleaning that exhibits characteristic [iv]) may be satisfactorily described as fears of, or discomfort about, some external object or situation, in contrast to the other OCD symptoms discussed earlier. Staying with this notion of an external object or situation, however, it is possible to formulate in these terms a theme shared by all of the various kinds of OCD symptoms identified in this discussion. All of those symptoms that, in contrast to phobic states, cannot be described as fears of, or discomfort about, external objects or situations can also be said, more vaguely, to involve a *different role* for external objects and situations than do phobic states – this more vague statement clearly follows from the less vague. But this more vague statement is applicable to the three kinds of OCD symptoms that can be described as fears of, or discomfort about, external objects or situations. Patients with symptoms that exhibit characteristic (v) and patients who exhibit the repetitive cleaning that exhibits characteristic (iv) do not remove themselves from, and do not have to have anything removed from, their environment in order to reduce their discomfort – the repetitive cleaners act to remove germs that are not actually present at all; patients suffering from symptoms exhibiting characteristic (v) merely rearrange their surroundings without removing anything from them. The actions of both kinds of patients are therefore in clear contrast to the behaviour undertaken by the phobic patient, which will involve either his removing himself from some fear-provoking situation or his having someone remove the phobic object from that situation.

The role played by external objects and situations in some of the symptoms that exhibit characteristic (iii) is perhaps closest to the role played in phobic states. Yet even in superstitious and bizarre thinking, the OCD patient's concerns are what might be termed "more remote" from the situations that provoke them than are the phobic's. Take, for example, the case where the patient removes small stones from pathways for fear that someone may trip on them. OCD symptoms of this kind involve the exercise of a great deal more "imagination" concerning possible dangers in the patient's situation than do the far less unlikely outcomes that disturb phobic patients. To this extent, therefore, one may once again assert that the role of external objects or situations in this kind of symptom is different from that found in phobic states.

One can adopt an alternative approach to this issue of there being a different role for external objects and situations in the case of category (iii) symptoms as opposed to phobic states. This approach is suggested by the fact that the patient in the examples considered is able to remove or reposition *for himself* the stones and books that are the source of his fear or discomfort. His problem does not involve his being unable to touch or be near any object or his having to escape from, or avoid, any situation. Indeed, far from wanting to escape, the patient will feel obliged to remain in the situation that makes him uncomfortable so that he can neutralise what he perceives to be the danger within it. This, then, appears to be an entirely separate way in which this kind of OCD symptom features a different role for external objects and situations than do phobic states – the latter involving the patient's being unable to be near certain things or having to escape from, or avoid, certain situations.

Indeed, a number of the other types of OCD symptoms involve a different role for external objects and situations than do phobic states. Category (v) symptoms and at least much of the repetitive checking in category (iv) do not usually involve the patient's having to escape or avoid anything, nor his being unable to be near to, or touch, some object. These symptoms, therefore, can be said to feature a different role for external objects or situations in this way, as well as in those ways identified earlier.

It needs finally to be noted that still other types of OCD symptoms do involve the patient's having to escape from, or avoid, certain situations. Those symptoms in category (i) that feature unacceptable impulses, for example, will usually involve the patient's being unable to bear being in (and thus having to escape from or avoid) certain situations – that is, those that provoke his impulses.

To sum up this discussion of the distinction between phobic states and OCD, it has been pointed out that, in a variety of ways, OCD symptoms can be distinguished from phobic states in featuring what may be termed a different role for external objects and situations from that played by such objects and situations in phobic states. The foregoing discussion has been restricted to this OCD–phobias distinction and says nothing as to how OCD might be distinguished from non-phobic disorders such as, for example, depressive illnesses or other anxiety disorders (although note the comments in Section 1.3.2). Some remarks concerning disorders that involve delusions will be made later.

1.3.7 The criterion of senselessness

It has been explicitly stated in the foregoing discussion that each of the features considered is not sufficient for those symptoms that exhibit it to be classifiable as OCD. These features are sufficient to distinguish OCD symptoms from phobic states, but this leaves open the question of whether or not any of these features are shared by some nonphobic phenomena that are not instances of OCD. The question of what else might be required to justify a diagnosis of OCD was earlier set to one side as unnecessary for an account of the distinction between OCD and phobic states.

The question is, nonetheless, one worth paying a little attention to, as it has some bearing on the critique of the traditional diagnostic criteria for OCD offered earlier (see Section 1.2.6). Consider again those OCD fears that concern the exercise of one's own will. This experience of fearing how one may act is clearly not by itself sufficient to justify a diagnosis of OCD. Plainly, there are instances of people's feeling scared about what they might intentionally do or of their experiencing impulses to do things they find unacceptable, without these experiences' being either OCD symptoms or their subclinical equivalents. As a result of extreme anger with another person, for example, someone might say that she is scared of the harm she thinks she might do to that person. This experience is readily distinguishable from that reported by the OCD patient – especially if the angry person's fear concerns only later regrets she may have, or legal punishments she may face as a result of her doing harm to another, while her immediate impulse is quite unequivocally to act in precisely this manner. It seems that the feature of senselessness is required with symptoms of this kind before they begin to take on an OCD aspect. The very desire to do harm must itself strike the patient as inappropriate or alien. (Note that resistance is not so important to this distinction – the angry person in the aforementioned example may resist her aggressive impulses merely by virtue of her fear of later regrets or legal sanction.)

It was argued in Section 1.2.6 that there are some OCD symptoms – the rituals of many of these patients, for example – that are not experienced as senseless and that this feature is thus not necessary for a diagnosis of OCD. Placing OCD symptoms such as these rituals side by side with those symptoms involving aggressive impulses, one can clearly see that the role of senselessness in the diagnosis of OCD is similar to that of characteristics (i)–(v). That is, although it plays no part in defining some symptoms as OCD, senselessness is crucial in defining other symptoms as such. Senselessness, however, may also be contrasted with the five characteristics discussed earlier, in that it does not form any part of the OCD–phobic states distinction. Aggressive impulses, that is, are not phobic symptoms whether or not they are experienced as senseless.

1.3.8   *The distinction between obsessional and psychotic thinking*

Reed (1985, p. 9) argues that the absence of reported insight in psychotic delusions means that obsessions may be "readily differentiated" from them. He suggests that deluded subjects, by definition, "lack insight [and find] nothing strange or senseless in their often palpably absurd ideas". As Reed puts it, the distinction between delusions and obsessions is a matter of form rather than content – it is a matter of how the patient thinks about something (the degree of insight he exhibits, for example) rather than what he thinks about, according to Reed.

Snaith also points out that "the theme of the retention of insight into the morbid nature of the idea" has been traditionally seen as central to the distinction between a neurotic and a psychotic symptom (1981, p. 85). He goes on to quote Kraüpl-Taylor, who makes a most interesting contribution in tracing this distinction back to demonological theories and "the distinction between *possession* and *obsession*; in the latter, the evil spirits surround the individual (Latin: *obsidere*, to besiege), whereas in possession the spirit enters into its victim and dominates him completely" (Snaith, 1981, p. 85, original emphasis). Thus, "possession" is presented as the counterpart of the modern notion of *delusion,* where this notion – in contrast, it is claimed, to the state of being obsessed – is understood to involve necessarily the patient's having no insight into the morbidity of his thinking. It consists, that is, of his having been completely "taken over" by his morbid thinking.

Yet the critique of the standard diagnostic criteria for OCD (Section 1.2.6) suggests that, contrary to Reed's position and the traditional account of neurotic pathology outlined by Snaith, the absence of reported insight cannot distinguish all obsessions from delusions. Although it has already been noted that senselessness is indeed crucial in defining some symptoms as OCD, this feature is not shared by all instances of the disorder.

Further difficulties for Reed's position may be raised by those patients who are classified by some diagnosticians as "partially deluded". These patients are held to have beliefs that would otherwise satisfy the criteria for delusions but do not hold these beliefs with absolute conviction: "partial delusions are expressed with doubt, as a possibility which the subject entertains but is not certain about" (Wing et al., quoted in Garety, 1985, p. 29).

1.3.9 A content-based distinction between obsessions and partial delusions/delusions?

How, then, are obsessions to be distinguished from partial delusions, and how are those cases of OCD where reported insight is absent to be distinguished from delusions? Perhaps this is, in Reed's terms, sometimes a matter of the content, rather than the form, of the patient's thinking, contrary to Reed's suggestion.

Consider Mullen's (1979) approach to the definition of delusions, which has been described as "representative of present-day British and American views" (Garety, 1985, p. 29). Mullen appears to agree with Reed in some measure when, early on in his discussion, he says that "a delusion is...judged to be present more from the manner in which it is adhered to [that is, its *form* in Reed's terms] and the reason for its emergence than any aspect of content" (Mullen, 1979, p. 29). Mullen also notes, however, that this distinction between form and content is easier to maintain regarding disorders of perception than disorders of belief, and he goes on to include, among other characteristics "usually attributed" to delusions, that "their *content* is often fantastic or at least inherently unlikely" (Mullen, 1979, p. 36, emphasis not in original). (Mullen also notes that a true belief may be a delusion, and this might at first be thought to conflict with his criterion of the belief's being fantastic or inherently unlikely – but such a case might presumably still meet this criterion by the true belief's being held for bizarre reasons.)

Regarding the question of the distinction between delusions and obsessions, Mullen himself, like Reed, regards the "formal" characteristics of the patient's thinking as crucial. But because such characteristics have already been questioned, how successfully might this distinction be instead drawn, contrary to Mullen's own account, in terms of his characterisation of the contents of delusions ?

Two points suggest that Mullen's content-based criterion would not be sufficiently specific to distinguish delusions from obsessions. Firstly, as has already been argued, at least some obsessions seem to have bizarre contents, and indeed, very many seem to involve a concern for, at best, inherently unlikely matters. Secondly, DSM-III-R distinguishes between bizarre and nonbizarre delusions, the latter "involving situations that occur in real life, such as being followed, poisoned, infected, loved at a distance, being deceived by one's spouse or lover" (DSM-III-R, p. 202). This evidently amounts to a denial that all delusions have to be fantastic or inherently unlikely, and it may therefore be concluded that Mullen's content-based criterion could not be used to distinguish obsessions from delusions – some obsessions appear to meet this criterion whereas some delusions do not. (However, see the remarks earlier in this section regarding delusions that involve true beliefs; a delusion the content of which is not bizarre might nonetheless be believed on grounds that are – unless, of course, the content of a belief is understood to include the grounds on which it is held.)

1.3.10 Ego boundaries

Can more specific contents than those mentioned by Mullen be used to distinguish some delusions from obsessions? What if one considers only the type of thinking that DSM-III-R defines as *bizarre delusions* – for example, the belief that thoughts are being removed from one's mind (*thought withdrawal*), the belief that thoughts that are not one's own are being inserted into one's mind (*thought insertion*), and the belief that one's thoughts, as they occur, are being broadcast from one's mind to the external world so that others can hear them (*thought broadcasting*)? All of these examples share the theme of the patient's ego boundaries' being blurred – his own mental states are misidentified as public phenomena and/or as belonging to somebody else. Are these ego boundary confusions sufficient for the person who suffers them to be both (1) not diagnosable as OCD and (2) diagnosable as deluded – or at least as partially deluded should this confusion be expressed as a possibility rather than a certainty?

It is the question of whether or not bizarre thinking of the "blurred ego boundary" variety is sufficient to disqualify a person's thinking as being symptomatic of OCD that is of most relevance to the present discussion. A patient included in a study by the author (Jakes, 1992, Chapters 2, 5, and 6) and who was diagnosed as OCD shows that it is possible for a patient exhibiting certain kinds of ego boundary confusion to receive this diagnosis. (The patient does not exhibit either thought insertion or thought broadcasting, so her case does not count against the suggestion that these forms of ego boundary confusion are sufficient to rule out an OCD diagnosis.) D.S. was a 29-year-old woman whose major fear was that unwanted "obscene" thoughts she had might travel from her head, down her arms, and out of her body onto objects she was touching, and she would be punished for having left these thoughts on these objects. This situation she described as her thoughts' "contaminating" the objects. She reported that she often tried not to think, or to stop thinking, about her thoughts leaving her body (that is, she resisted these ideas of her thoughts leaving her body), but was ambivalent as to the morbidity of this way of thinking (that is, her reported insight was at most partial). Her response to thinking that her thoughts had contaminated objects was to repeat (up to fifty times) whatever she had been doing – for example, getting up out of a chair – at the time the contamination was supposed to have taken place. This, she reported, would eventually erase the thought from her mind, and she would then think that this thought had also been removed from the object it had been contaminating.

Although it might be argued that the diagnosis this woman was given was questionable, how, working on the tentative assumption that it is correct, might one seek to justify it? Why, in particular, should this woman not be diagnosed as being at least partially deluded? Is this not supported by the content of her thinking having the theme it does, while she expresses some (but by no means complete) insight into the morbidity of this thinking?

Against a diagnosis of "partially deluded", is it perhaps the behaviour of this patient – her repetitive action intended by some magical means to undo harm thought by her to have occurred (behaviour, that is, which exhibits characteristics [iii] and [iv]) – that makes her diagnosable as OCD? And if she were to report the very same thinking – a half-doubted fear that her thoughts had escaped and were contaminating surrounding objects – in the absence of any repeated action, would the OCD diagnosis not then seem inappropriate, and a "partially deluded" or "deluded" diagnosis far more likely be correct? On this argument, the patient's symptoms can be distinguished from bizarre delusions (or bizarre partial delusions), but not on the grounds of either the form or the content of her thinking. It is being tentatively suggested that her thinking can thus not be distinguished at all from such deluded or partially deluded states when considered in isolation from its behavioural consequences.

Another example may help to argue the same conclusion. Reed (1985, p. 141) presents two patients – "Mr E", whose everyday life was severely constricted by his fear about the insidious spread of germs, disease and corruption; and "Mr A", who harboured fears of identical content. The former patient is described by Reed as having an obsession, the latter a delusion of the "nihilistic" variety, as is not uncommonly observed in depressive disorders. The fact that "Mr E" resists his thoughts, Reed suggests, is crucial to this distinction, but Reed cannot be correct here because, as has been argued in Section 1.2.6.2, some OCD patients do not resist obsessions that are otherwise very like those this patient reports.

Among other grounds on which such a nihilistic delusion might be distinguished from obsessions with similar contents is, arguably, the behavioural consequences of the patient's thinking. Thus, some depressed patients say that they regard the world as full of disease and contamination, but it is only when a patient responds to this thinking by resorting to soap and scrubbing brushes to protect himself and/or others that it is perhaps at least more likely that an alternative or additional diagnosis will be OCD.

It must once again be stressed that these tentative suggestions amount to no more than the claim that *some* obsessions can be distinguished from delusions by the behaviour that they provoke. The necessity for this restriction to only *some* obsessions is most obviously argued by the fact that in certain cases obsessions may provoke no compulsive behaviour at all and could, by virtue of this, scarcely be either characterised as obsessions or distinguished from delusions. Other criteria must be at work in these cases, with some of the other features examined in the case of the phobia–OCD distinction – for example, characteristics (i) and (ii) – perhaps sometimes playing a role in distinguishing the patient's thinking from delusional states.

A picture similar to that observed in the case of the phobia–OCD distinction already begins to emerge here, therefore. There is no one way, or single dimension in terms of which, delusions and obsessions may be distinguished. There are various ways, with features (such as repetitive behaviour) that are not common to all cases of OCD once again sometimes playing a part in distinguishing some obsessions from delusions.

1.3.11   Summary and discussion

It has been suggested that the existing defining criteria for OCD are inadequate, that there is no single set of features both common and peculiar to all instances of the disorder, and that there is no single way in which OCD may be distinguished from phobic or delusional states; a number of different ways in which these distinctions between OCD and other states may be drawn have been noted.

The approach to the definition of OCD that has been defended here, in suggesting that no single set of features is both common and peculiar to all instances of the disorder, is similar to the definition of schizophrenia offered by DSM-III-R. That definition suggests that a person may receive a diagnosis of schizophrenia when *any one* of features (i), (ii) or (iii) is present (all quotes from DSM-III-R, p. 194):

(i)   "two of the following: (a) delusions, (b) prominent hallucinations, (c) incoherence or marked loosening of associations, (d) catatonic behaviour, (e) flat or grossly inappropriate affect"
(ii)   "bizarre delusions"

(iii) "prominent hallucinations", involving, for example, "a voice keeping up a running commentary on the person's behaviour or thoughts"

Thus, features that are not common to all of the patients who receive a diagnosis of schizophrenia may be sufficient, when present, for this diagnosis to be made. More generally, the introduction to DSM-III-R (p. xxiv) draws a distinction between *monothetic* and *polythetic* diagnostic criteria – in the former, each of several features must be present for a diagnosis to be made; in the latter, a list of diagnostic features is given, *a certain number, but not necessarily all,* of which must be present for a diagnosis to be made. Although the approach to the definition of OCD offered here may differ considerably from the standard defining criteria for the disorder, this approach does not represent a radical departure from all existing diagnostic practice. Its central claim is that OCD is identified, like schizophrenia (and a number of other diagnostic categories), on the basis of polythetic criteria (also see Cooper and Cooper, 1988, p. 9).

The present discussion is concerned only with the definition of OCD – there is no suggestion that this definition's subdivisions of OCD symptoms are important from the point of view of such matters as the explanation or treatment of the disorder. It is too early to claim any such importance for these subdivisions, and indeed any differences among OCD patients in terms of the aetiology and/or treatment of their disorder may turn out to be unrelated to differences in the kinds of symptoms they report (also see Chapter 8).

2   Behavioural/learning accounts of OCD

2.1   An outline of the model

The behavioural/learning account of OCD (e.g., Eysenck and Rachman, 1965) is based on Mowrer's (1939,1960) "two factor" theory of learning. This approach provides very similar accounts of both OCD and phobic states. The preoccupations of OCD patients are held by this approach to concern feared stimuli that have acquired anxiety-producing properties by a process of classical conditioning. The behavioural/learning account suggests that the compulsions provoked by these feared stimuli are escape or avoidance behaviour. According to this account, this behaviour reduces or prevents anxiety and is thus reinforced by a process of instrumental conditioning. De Silva (1988) suggests that "the model is essentially one of learned anxiety reduction". In the case of OCD, as in the case of phobias, the avoidance behaviour may be passive (for example, not approaching objects thought to be contaminated) or active (for example, checking for contamination [Gray, 1982, p. 440]). An example of an OCD escape behaviour is cleaning to remove what is thought to be some contamination.

The model is not substantially altered by the recognition that it is not only anxiety but also other forms of mood disturbance, subsumed under the vaguer term "discomfort" (Rachman and Hodgson, 1980), that is reported by some OCD patients. The maintenance of compulsions is then attributed to learned discomfort reduction (de Silva, 1988).

Consistent with this account, Rachman and his co-workers (e.g., Hodgson and Rachman, 1972; Rachman, de Silva, and Roper, 1976; Rachman and Hodgson, 1980) have shown that compulsions are indeed often provoked by environmental cues, and that when OCD patients are exposed to these cues they experience an increase in anxiety or discomfort. These workers have also shown that when these patients carry out their compulsive behaviour, they often experience a considerable reduction in discomfort. This is cited by de Silva (1988) as support for the behavioural/learning model, as are the results of behaviour therapy with the disorder.

2.2   Preparedness and incubation

Eysenck (1979) has proposed a number of modifications of the behavioural/learning model in the light of several difficulties, including the following:

(a) The *selectivity* of the stimuli that elicit fear and discomfort in OCD and phobic states is not explained. Far from being a largely random sample as the model predicts, some stimuli are greatly overrepresented in OCD and phobic states (e.g., dirt and spiders), whereas others, which seem very likely to be sometimes associated with aversive stimuli (e.g., cars and guns), seem to be underrepresented.

(b) In a large number of cases, there is no evidence that the stimuli that elicit fear and discomfort in OCD and phobic states have been paired, let alone repeatedly paired, with aversive stimuli at the onset of the disorder.

(c) The stimuli that elicit fear and discomfort in OCD and phobic states do not undergo extinction despite their presentation's being unaccompanied by aversive stimuli.

Eysenck (1979) attempts to meet these difficulties by supplementing the behavioural/learning model with the concepts of *preparedness* (Seligman, 1971) and *incubation*. According to the preparedness hypothesis, some stimuli more readily acquire aversive associations because of the evolutionary advantage these associations are postulated to have bestowed. It would be suggested, for example, that a fear of spiders or snakes has conferred such an advantage by producing avoidance of life-threatening members of these species. It would be similarly argued that phylogenetically novel stimuli that are connected with genuine dangers (e.g., cars and guns) do not appear in OCD and phobic states because they have had no opportunity to become "prepared". It is, this, then, that explains the selectivity of the fear/discomfort-eliciting cues seen in OCD and phobic states and thus meets difficulty (a), according to Eysenck.

It is less clear what Eysenck's account has to say concerning difficulty (b). Perhaps prepared stimuli could be hypothesised to acquire numerous *mildly* aversive associations that summate to produce clinical levels of discomfort. In addition or alternatively, it might be hypothesised that clinical levels of discomfort are reached because *mildly* aversive associations are subject to incubation. In both of these hypotheses, an attempt is made to explain how OCD (and phobic states) can arise without the stimuli that are involved in these disorders having been paired with stimuli that are *highly* aversive. But again, in the case of either of these hypotheses, the account would require the stimuli that are involved in these disorders always to have been paired with stimuli that are to some extent aversive. It may be doubted, therefore, whether difficulty (b) has really been answered at all.

Eysenck's incubation hypothesis, which states that the fear/discomfort elicited by a conditioned stimulus may be augmented, rather than extinguished, by unaccompanied presentations of that stimulus thus attempts to answer difficulty (c). A number of objections have been brought against the incubation hypothesis. Bersch (1980) argues that the evidence for incubation is very limited and that, at its present stage of development, the concept in any case lacks predictive power; this objection is echoed by Gray (1979). Bersch thus concludes that the "contribution [of the concept of incubation] to an understanding of 'paradoxical' failures of extinction [and] the etiology of neuroses [i.e., difficulties (c) and (b) here respectively] must remain in doubt" (Bersch, 1980, p. 16).

2.3   The anxiety reduction hypothesis

As noted earlier, de Silva (1988) cites as support for the behavioural/learning model the finding that anxiety/discomfort is often reduced by compulsive behaviour. As de Silva also notes, however, in some cases compulsions fail to reduce, and may even increase, the patient's anxiety/discomfort. This is especially true of those patients in whose compulsions checking behaviour predominates (Rachman and Hodgson, 1980).

Rachman and Hodgson (1980) suggest that anxiety/discomfort-increasing checking rituals are reinforced by their long-term consequences – for example, the avoidance of future disasters that the patient perceives the rituals to confer. This is despite the increase in discomfort associated with these compulsions in the short term, which the long-term benefits are argued by Rachman and Hodgson to counterbalance. But it is precisely the difficulty of ascertaining whether or not any such long-term benefits have been produced that Rachman and Hodgson also use, as will be seen, to explain the doubting, repetitiveness, and low levels of anxiety/discomfort-reduction that are associated with checking compulsions. These authors can surely not have it both ways.

The behavioural/learning view that anxiety/discomfort-decreasing compulsions are maintained because of the patient's experience in carrying out these compulsions – that is, due to "learned anxiety reduction" – may in any event be mistaken. This account appears to assimilate such behaviour too closely to that of animals in learning experiments (see de Silva, 1988, for some examples of animal learning studies that he points out have been "cited as possibly relevant to OCD" [p. 207]). The consequences of carrying out some behaviour (e.g., lever pressing) in a laboratory task are indeed often the major factor that may be expected to control a laboratory animal's performance of the behaviour. But much of the compulsive cleaning and checking of OCD patients, for example, may be contrasted with such animal behaviour in this respect. Thus, the belief that cleaning something will make it less contaminated or that checking something ensures that it is not in a dangerous state is shared by normals and OCD patients alike. In the case of OCD patients, these beliefs are, therefore, unlikely to be supported only by the patients' experience in carrying out cleaning or checking compulsions, for example – it is reasonable to suppose, that is, that OCD patients will hold these beliefs at least in part for the same reasons that normals do. These beliefs provide a reason for cleaning something thought to be contaminated or checking something thought to be a possible source of danger. An OCD patient has, in consequence, a reason for carrying out many cleaning or checking compulsions that is independent of the effects of these compulsions on his level of discomfort. It should be no surprise, therefore, that – contrary to the anxiety reduction hypothesis – some anxiety/discomfort-increasing compulsions are maintained; it can be further suggested that – contrary to the behavioural/learning view – the anxiety/discomfort reduction brought about by the performance of many compulsions is not a major factor in maintaining the performance of these compulsions. On the present view, that is, patients will usually clean things simply because they think that these things are contaminated and that cleaning them will make them less contaminated. Similarly, they will usually check things because they think that these things may be in a state that presents a source of danger and that checking them will ascertain whether or not this is the case. Discomfort reduction may well frequently result from the performance of such cleaning and checking behaviour but is not necessary for an explanation of the performance or maintenance of such behaviour.

2.4 Behaviour therapy

De Silva (1988) also cites "the numerous treatment studies of obsessive-compulsive patients using the exposure–response prevention paradigm" (p. 205; e.g., Emmelkamp, 1982; Foa, Steketee, and Ozarow, 1985) as support for the behavioural/learning approach that helped to inspire the use of this paradigm with OCD. It has been argued, however, that many of the suggestions made by behaviour therapists as regards the remediation of OCD were anticipated by Janet (Pitman, 1987a, 1987b; Cottraux, 1990) on the basis of a quite different model of OCD, although some objections to this interpretation of Janet's are offered elsewhere (see Section 4.7.3). The mechanisms by which exposure with response prevention may work with OCD continue to be a matter for debate. Many, or even most, accounts of the disorder are able to provide some explanation for why this treatment should be effective with the disorder. Thus, although the effects of exposure with response prevention have been explained in terms of conditioning mechanisms (Eysenck, 1979), accounts of these effects have also been offered in terms of innate fear mechanisms (Gray, 1979, 1982), "perceptions of self-efficacy" (Bandura, 1978; Southworth and Kirsch, 1988) and various other alternatives (for example, see Sections 3.5, 4.7.3, 6.7, and 8.2). Although it might be argued that any theory of OCD must be able to make sense of the effects of exposure therapy with response prevention with the disorder, being able to do so cannot in itself be strong support for that theory. It should also be noted that there are some authors who would dispute just how effective exposure with response prevention has been shown to be in treating OCD, mainly on the grounds of what these authors suggest to be design flaws in the treatment outcome studies (for example, Montgomery, 1990). Such objections do seem to apply to early investigations of exposure with response prevention with OCD patients, such as Rachman, Hodgson, and Marks (1971), Hodgson, Rachman, and Marks (1972), and Roper et al. (1975). (See Emmelkamp, 1982, Chapter 8, for a full discussion of these studies.) All of these studies failed to counterbalance their treatments; all of the patients who were included received control treatments, such as relaxation and modelling, before receiving exposure with response prevention, making the comparison of this treatment with the control procedures very difficult, if not impossible. Such flaws do not exist, however, in the study of exposure with response prevention by Marks et al. (1980), which does indeed show this treatment to be more effective for OCD patients than a relaxation procedure. (See Marks, 1981, pp. 45–75, for a discussion of this and other OCD treatment outcome studies.)

2.5   The repetitiveness of some compulsive behaviour

Gray (1982, p. 441) suggests that the learning/behavioural model fails to explain why compulsive behaviours occur repetitively and suggests that a common explanation for this and the repetitiveness of obsessions should be sought. It is necessary to qualify this criticism because, as Rachman and Hodgson (1980) note, not all compulsive behaviours are performed repetitively. These authors, as noted earlier, distinguish those patients ("cleaners") among whom cleaning compulsions predominate from those ("checkers") among whom checking compulsions predominate and report that, as compared with cleaners, checkers tend to exhibit (a) more repetitiveness in their rituals, (b) more doubts as to how effective their rituals have been, and (c) less relief from discomfort/anxiety from their rituals. According to Rachman and Hodgson but against Gray, therefore, it is not the repetitiveness of compulsive behaviours per se, but rather the repetitiveness of checking compulsions that stands in need of explanation.

Having drawn these three distinctions between checkers and cleaners, Rachman and Hodgson go on to offer an explanation of the distinctions in terms of the nature of the tasks involved in checking and cleaning difficulties. Thus, cleaners are trying, it is suggested, to remove a source of discomfort that is "already present and usually evident (visually or tactually)", whereas checkers, by contrast, are trying to reduce the probability of aversive future events (for example, the consequences of leaving lights on and plugs in sockets). Final confirmation as to the outcome of rituals, Rachman and Hodgson argue, is therefore more easily available to cleaners than to checkers, and this, they say, explains both (1) why checkers tend to show repetition, doubting and low levels of relief as regards their compulsions and (2) why their compulsions exhibit these features to a greater extent than do those of cleaners.

A number of objections may be brought against this account. Firstly, if cleaners are thought to be scared of illness and so on, which is regarded by them as the likely result of not cleaning well enough, future consequences are involved here as much as they are in the case of checkers. Rachman and Hodgson would perhaps answer this point by arguing that cleaners have a fear of dirt rather than of the consequences of not removing dirt. Quite apart from the entirely post hoc character of this reply, however, it is doubtful that it succeeds in rendering final confirmation more available to cleaners. Is it, for example, harder to make certain that all the plugs are out of their sockets in a room than it is to make certain that every last particle of dirt has been removed from one's hands? If anything, it should be easier to be certain that plugs are out, especially when one considers the notion of dirt and germs one cannot see, as stressed, for example, by adverts for soap powders.

But the checker knows, it might be objected, that even if all the plugs are out and switches are off, it is possible that the future events he is trying to avoid – his house burning down, for one – may still occur. This is true, but is not a good explanation of why the checker has doubts about, and repeats, his compulsions. If the feared future consequences may still occur despite plugs' being out, and if this is what preys on the checker's mind, it gives him no reason to doubt, and repeat, his checks. Such fears would, if anything, lead him into checking other things – for example, fuse boxes, after he has checked plugs. Thus, although Rachman and Hodgson's account may be able to make sense of the low levels of relief reported by checkers, one must conclude that neither the tendency of checkers to have doubts about, and to repeat, their compulsions, nor their tendency to do these things to a greater extent than do cleaners, has been satisfactorily explained.

De Silva (1988) refers to Teasdale's (1974) discussion for an explanation of the repetitiveness of compulsions. De Silva follows Teasdale in arguing "that compulsive behaviours may be considered as avoidance behaviours which are under poor stimulus control" (de Silva, 1988, p. 206). He suggests that these behaviours do not have "good feedback or safety signal properties" (p. 206) and that it is their lacking these properties that explains their repetitiveness. De Silva makes this suggestion as regards both cleaning and checking compulsions. Yet, if the earlier arguments are accepted, it is precisely the compulsions to which these points would seem to be most applicable – that is, those involving cleaning behaviours – that tend not to be repeatedly performed. Couching the earlier arguments in de Silva's terms, it is the poor detectability of possible sources of contamination that appear to render the compulsive cleaner's task one with poor "feedback" or "safety signals", yet it is compulsive checkers who tend to repeat their behaviour.

The compulsive checker's task might also, as de Silva suggests, be argued to have poor feedback or safety signals. This is a restatement of the earlier claim that the possible future consequences the patient is trying to avoid may still occur despite, for example, all plugs' being out and all switches off. But for the same reasons as those previously offered, this cannot explain why checking compulsions tend to be repeated. That is, the patient has, in de Silva's terms, perfectly good feedback or safety signals as regards the immediate outcome of those actions he repeats. It is, objectively speaking, easy to establish whether or not plugs have been removed or switches turned off, and the patient's repetitive behaviour cannot be explained by the uncertain nature of – or the poor feedback or safety signals he has with respect to – longer-term outcomes.

2.6 Obsessions that are not provoked by environmental cues

As was previously noted, the behavioural/learning approach provides very similar accounts of both OCD and phobic states. What, then, of those obsessions that, unlike phobic fear (and many obsessions), are not provoked by any environmental stimuli at all? Examples of obsessions that might not be so provoked are

(a) images of horribly mutilated dead bodies,
(b) blasphemous thoughts,
(c) unacceptable insults concerning, for example, the appearance or conduct of the patient's partner or close relatives, and
(d) number sequences and nonsense phrases that continually run through the patient's mind.

(See Section 1.3.4.3 for a discussion of a closely related feature – the fear/discomfort in such obsessions having a covert object – as one of the criteria by which OCD is *by definition* distinguished from phobic states.)

All of these obsessions that are not provoked by environmental cues may trouble the patient in any place or at any time. The occurrence of such obsessions, that is, may not be associated with the patient's having been or being in any particular kind of situation, such as having had contact with what the patient thinks to be some contaminating material or being in the presence of any specific person. Such environmental provocations may, of course, exist for some cases of obsessions like those listed in the opening of this section; all that is being claimed is that environmental provocations do not exist for *all* such cases.

Rachman (1978) provides an analysis of obsessions in general that may be applied to obsessions of this kind in particular. This analysis emphasises the similarities between obsessions, which are termed in this analysis "noxious [internal] stimuli to which patients fail to habituate" (p. 264), and phobic objects. Rachman suggests that obsessions, like phobic objects, give rise to anxiety and overt or covert escape and avoidance behaviour and may even be accompanied by physiological reactions similar to those elicited by phobic stimuli.

In the case of some obsessions, not all of these hypothesised similarities to phobic objects hold good. Thus, as Rachman and Hodgson themselves note (1980, p. 274), the analysis "provides little enlightenment about silly, insignificant obsessions such as number sequences, nonsensical phrases and the like" (refer back to example [d]). It seems in such cases more likely to be the patient's frustration at having such trivial matter on his mind (and less likely to be provoked anxiety) that is at the heart of his distress, contrary to Rachman's (1978) analysis. This difficulty for the behavioural/learning approach may also arise in the case of some obsessions that, in contrast to those in question at present, are provoked by environmental cues (although see Salkovskis, 1985, for an attempt to explain such cases within an approach broadly similar to Rachman's).

But what of those cases where obsessions do exhibit the similarities stressed in Rachman's analysis, as is likely to be the case in examples (a)–(c)? Some objections are offered by Gray (1982). He argues that these "cognitive phenomena [obsessions] are not behaviour" but are, rather, "part of the systems that control behaviour". To suppose that these systems follow the same laws as behaviour is, Gray suggests, "the same kind of mistake as the belief that the neural display on the visual cortex is inspected by a second pair of eyes" (p. 441). Gray also argues that "if we treat internal events as behaviour, would we not expect noxious thoughts to be avoided passively, that is, not occur?"

Gray's first objection can probably be rejected. Any explanation of the functioning of the visual system in terms of "a second pair of eyes inside the head" would fail by leading to an infinite regress (Ryle, 1949). Rachman's analysis implies no infinite regress.

Gray's second objection states that Rachman's model treats internal events as behaviour, and yet it is, contrary to this objection, the supposed similarities between obsessions and external stimuli, not behaviour, that are stressed by Rachman's analysis. Nonetheless, Gray's objection introduces the important issue of how the occurrence of obsessions of the type in question is to be explained by Rachman's model. Thus, it seems that any account that models obsessions on phobic stimuli cannot hope to illuminate the question of why obsessions of this kind occur at all. De Silva (1988) refers to this question as a "relatively neglected aspect of obsessive-compulsive disorder" (p. 212). A patient's experiencing an obsession is supposed, on Rachman's account, to be analogous to a phobic patient's encountering his feared environmental cues. Yet how the phobic patient encounters these feared cues – how, that is, his episodes of fear occur – is unproblematic. This is simply a matter of the patient's being *in a certain kind of place* or in contact with *a certain environmental cue*. Because of the very nature of obsessions of the kind in question, the occurrence of these obsessions cannot be explained in these terms.

This is not, of course, the only basis on which the value of Rachman's model can be assessed. Its value can also be judged, for example, in respect to the treatment suggestions to which the model gives rise, this being the aspect of Rachman's contribution that has been most energetically followed up. The model has been presented as a rationale for using – for obsessions of the type in question – treatments that are adapted from the existing behavioural treatments for phobias (and treatments for obsessions that are provoked by external cues). Therefore, those working under Rachman's influence have directed their efforts to devising treatments for these obsessions that involve exposure to the patient's "noxious internal stimuli" while preventing the performance of any associated anxiety-reducing compulsions. Most recently, the approach that has been adopted in the attempt to provide such a treatment is to play for patients the contents of their obsessional thoughts, recorded on 30-second loop-tapes in the patients' own voices.

The support that the results from this approach have so far provided for Rachman's model is at best equivocal. Thus, although there are a few promising single-case reports in which this intervention has been used (Headland and McDonald, 1987; Salkovskis and Westbrook, 1989), Lovell et al. (1991) report the first controlled investigation of the intervention – a small study with six patients in each of two groups. In this study, the intervention was compared with a control treatment in that patients were played recordings (once again in the patients' own voices) of "neutral nonaxiogenic material" – that is, material (such as passages of poetry) that was unconnected with the contents of the patient's obsessions. No significant differences between the effects of these two types of tape were found after eight weeks of treatment.

These authors also note, however, that four of the patients in the experimental group improved, as opposed to only one in the control group; these four experimental patients were those who found the taped contents of their obsessional thoughts anxiogenic. Despite the absence of any significant difference between the two groups in Lovell et al.'s study, therefore, their results provide, as these authors note, some indication that recordings of the contents of obsessions may be a useful intervention for at least some patients. Further research is plainly required here, and it must meanwhile be concluded that definite confirmation of the efficacy of this treatment, which Rachman's model helped to inspire, has yet to be provided.

2.7   Emotional processing

Attempts to explain obsessions as conditioned emotional responses and/or noxious internal stimuli to which patients have failed to habituate have been subjected to criticism here. De Silva (1988) goes elsewhere in the behavioural literature in order to find what he regards as "perhaps the best explanation for the persistence of obsessions, and of how normal intrusions become more chronic and achieve clinically significant levels of severity" (p. 212). This explanation is provided, de Silva suggests, by "the broad concept of emotional processing as proposed by Rachman".

Rachman (1980) introduces this concept of emotional processing in an attempt to help unify such apparently unrelated phenomena as obsessions, the return of fear, abnormal grief reactions and nightmares. Rachman acknowledges many dissimilarities between these phenomena. But he believes there to be a need to establish "unifying concepts", given that some fear-reducing procedures are able to produce comparable improvements in different forms of disorders – for example, exposure-based treatments for phobias, OCD and (possibly) abnormal grief reactions.

Another, quite separate, reason for introducing the concept of emotional processing is provided by Rachman. He suggests that although the undue persistence of fear (and therefore perhaps of obsessions, too) is open to numerous explanations, the unprovoked return of fear following a diminution presents difficulties for traditional theories. The return of fear implies that at least some of the original fear reduction must have been transient and thus, Rachman suggests, incompletely processed. This phenomenon of the return of fear occupies much of Rachman's discussion in his 1980 paper.

Rachman proposes that obsessions, nightmares, the return of fear and numerous other phenomena be treated as indices of "unsatisfactory emotional processing" and that therapies for these various conditions be formulated as attempts to facilitate the desired emotional processing.

Rachman is aware of the circularity of argument that may result from regarding phenomena such as the return of fear as both *resulting from* and being an *index of* unsatisfactory emotional processing. He believes this circularity can be avoided by his proposal to use "test probes" – presenting patients, following the diminution of their fear, with the stimuli that were formerly distressing for them. An independent measure of emotional processing is provided, Rachman suggests, by the degree of distress provoked by the presentations of these stimuli.

Rachman goes on to discuss factors that may give rise to difficulties in, and factors that may promote, emotional processing. Finally he raises a number of questions he believes to follow from the introduction of the concept of emotional processing.

It seems clear that, according to the most obvious interpretations, Rachman's remarks may be taken to represent a substantial departure from conditioning explanations of phenomena such as fear and obsessions. One is entitled to suppose that Rachman intends his analysis to be taken as such by the stress he places upon the return of fear – a phenomenon, he evidently believes, that is not explained by conditioning explanations.

What, then, does this analysis put in the place of conditioning explanations? It would seem, unfortunately, not very much. Although plainly aware of the danger of circularity in his argument, Rachman has failed to avoid it. In particular, it is unlikely that test probes can perform the function Rachman suggests. The return of fear is defined by him as "literally the reappearance of some degree of a fear that had undergone some diminution" (1980, p. 54). This surely implies that at the time this diminution was observed, the subject's response to Rachman's test probes would have been more favourable (that is, it would have involved less or no distress in response to the presentation of these probes) than it would following the return of fear – if this were not so, it is indeed unlikely that one would have been tempted to speak of a diminution of fear in the first place. The same applies to the three other indices of satisfactory emotional processing suggested by Rachman (1980, p. 55, Table 1): the decline of subjective distress, the reduction of disturbed behaviour and the return of routine behaviour (for example, concentration). Reduction in these indices would be necessary before we could speak of the patient's fear having diminished. One must therefore conclude that the unsatisfactory emotional processing that is reflected in the phenomenon of the return of fear can only be judged to be present (can only judged to have occurred) once fear has actually reappeared following a diminution. In other words, the concept of emotional processing in the form in that it is presented by Rachman fails to cast any light on the phenomenon of the return of fear.

But if this is true of the concept as applied to this phenomenon – the one singled out by Rachman as pointing to the need for such a concept – it is more clearly true of its other applications in Rachman's paper. The numerous factors listed as promoting or impeding emotional processing (1980, p. 57,Table 4) are, for the most part, those that are, as Rachman himself notes, "already familiar to behaviour therapists" (p. 57) as the favourable and unfavourable conditions in which to

carry out behaviour therapy – for example, long presentations and repeated practice (both favourable conditions), and excessively brief presentations and inadequate practice (both unfavourable). These conditions appear to be unified by
Rachman only to the extent that the same *term* – emotional processing – is used
in describing their effect. Similarly, most of the questions raised by Rachman at
the end of his paper could have been just as readily raised without reference to the
concept of emotional processing at all. For example, the question, "does [a subject's being engaged in a complex task when presented with a fearful stimulus]
impede or facilitate the emotional processing [that will occur]?" (p. 58) is simply
the question, "do such tasks effect the reduction in fear brought about by presenting fearful stimuli?" but with the introduction of the term *emotional processing*.

Obsessions are not discussed in Rachman's paper in any detail, and for this
reason it is not entirely clear from that paper what it is that obsessions are supposed to indicate is in need of "processing". Is it some experience separate from –
but hypothesised to give rise to – obsessions, or rather only the content of obsessions themselves? If the former, then a theory of the origin and persistence of
obsessions would only be provided if some account were offered of which experiences produce obsessions, and of the mechanisms by which these experiences
have this effect. No such account is provided, nor would it be provided merely by
describing as "emotional processing" the relationship between obsessions on the
one hand and some experience hypothesised to give rise to obsessions on the
other. If it is only the content of obsessions that needs processing, then it is once
again not an explanation of obsessions that is being provided, but rather only a different way of talking about their varying degrees of severity – "this obsession is
a sign of a good deal of unsatisfactorily processed emotion" being translatable,
that is, as "this obsession is severe and will need a good deal of therapy".

2.8   The cognitive-behavioural account of OCD

The cognitive-behavioural account of OCD (McFall and Wollersheim, 1979;
Salkovskis, 1985, 1989; Rachman, 1993) is presented as a development of
behavioural approaches to the disorder. Thus, although the cognitive-behavioural
account attempts to supplement these approaches through the application of
Beck's cognitive model of psychopathology to OCD (Beck, 1976; Beck, Emery,
and Greenberg, 1985), Salkovskis notes (1985, p. 577) that it also "owes much
to the previous 'anatomy of obsessions' proposed by Rachman (1978), and
makes many of the same assumptions".

When considering the discomfort and compulsive behaviour of OCD
patients, the cognitive-behavioural account, along with the behavioural
approaches considered earlier, continues to formulate compulsions as escape
and avoidance behaviour and to suggest that such behaviour is maintained by
the discomfort reduction it produces. However, as regards the manner in which
discomfort and compulsions (termed *neutralising* by this approach) are pro-

voked and the means by which discomfort and compulsions attain clinical levels of severity, the cognitive-behavioural account takes issue with some behavioural approaches. The cognitive-behavioural account suggests that discomfort and compulsive behaviour are not directly provoked by obsessions but are, rather, the result of how obsessions are "appraised" by OCD patients. It is suggested that the occurrence and content of obsessions are interpreted by OCD patients "as an indication that they [the patients] might be responsible for harm to themselves or others" (Salkovskis, 1989, p. 678). It is this appraisal, Salkovskis suggests (p. 678), that leads to an obsession's being "a source of discomfort and an imperative signal for action" for these patients, not the occurrence or content of obsessions per se. This appraisal in turn also leads to compulsive behaviour – to attempts, that is, on the part of OCD patients "both to suppress and to neutralise" obsessions, *neutralising* being "voluntarily initiated activity that is intended to have the effect of reducing the perceived responsibility" (Salkovskis, 1989, p. 678). This hypothesised reduction of perceived responsibility in turn produces a reduction in the patient's discomfort, according to Salkovskis, and it is this, he argues, that maintains the patient's neutralising behaviour. (An example of this process of neutralising would be provided by a mother who, after having obsessional thoughts of harming her children, reduced the anxiety provoked by these thoughts by replacing them with "good thoughts" of her children's being safe and well, and/or by removing objects with which she might harm her children.)

Salkovskis suggests that appraisals and neutralising behaviour not only maintain, but also in much the same way produce, OCD. Salkovskis notes that mild, relatively infrequent "normal obsessions" are reported by normal populations and are unaccompanied in these populations by serious disturbance of mood and coping (Rachman and de Silva, 1978). In vulnerable individuals, however, according to Salkovskis, even such normal obsessions will be appraised as an indication that the individual may be responsible for harm and as "an imperative signal for action". Thus, Salkovskis suggests that "obsessional problems will occur in individuals who are distressed by the occurrence of intrusions, and also believe the occurrence of such cognitions indicates personal responsibility for distressing harm unless corrective action is taken" (1989, p. 678). According to Salkovskis, people who respond in this way to their experience of normal obsessions inadvertently increase still further their sense of responsibility and distress at this experience; eventually, by these means, their sense of responsibility and distress, as well as the accompanying neutralising behaviour, reach clinical levels of severity. Some aspects of this account of how discomfort and compulsive behaviour reach clinical levels of severity are shared by Eysenck's (1979) incubation hypothesis (see Section 2.2.2).

Rachman, who adopts a line somewhat similar to Salkovskis's, suggests that "obsessions become unduly significant only to the extent that the affected person attaches special meaning to them". He argues that whereas "the majority of people dismiss or ignore their unwanted intrusive thoughts...once a person attaches important meaning to [them], they tend to become distressing and adhesive" (Rachman, 1993, p. 152).

A number of difficulties confront this approach, some of that have been discussed elsewhere (Jakes, 1989a, 1989b). The most important of these difficulties will be considered here. Those concerning the account this approach offers of the distress experienced by OCD patients will be considered first, followed by those concerning the analysis this account presents of the genesis of OCD.

2.8.1 *The distress experienced by* OCD *patients*

In presenting his version of the cognitive-behavioural account of OCD, Rachman (1993) discusses what he terms the "psychological fusion of...thought and...actions" (p. 151). This occurs, Rachman suggests, when patients consider their obsessions as "morally equivalent" to some forbidden behaviour that those obsessions concern (p. 152). Such a patient, for example, experiences thoughts or images of his doing or having done something unacceptable or experiences impulses to do that thing and, as a consequence, regards himself as no better than if he had actually done it. Rachman argues that this attitude is most apparent in cases involving obsessions with blasphemous, sexual or aggressive themes and is perhaps still more commonly observed when such obsessions are impulses, rather than thoughts or images – this being, he notes, due to impulses' being "a step closer to action" than thoughts or images (p. 152). Rachman may overstate his case in arguing that these patients regard as morally equivalent their obsessions, on the one hand, and violent or blasphemous behaviour on the other (R. Shafran, personal communication, 1992), but it does seem likely that at least part of the distress experienced by patients who suffer from aggressive, sexual or blasphemous obsessions sometimes consists of guilt produced by these obsessions.

To accept this is not, however, to accept that what distinguishes these OCD patients from the normal population is their propensity to respond in this manner to such obsessions. Why should one not suppose that anyone would be similarly inclined to think badly of themselves as a result of experiencing obsessional impulses (say to harm their relatives) with the frequency and intensity with which such impulses are experienced by those OCD patients for whom they are a major problem? On this objection, most people are not inclined to think badly of themselves simply because, not being OCD patients, if they experience any such obsessional impulses at all, these experiences will only be infrequent and not very intense. On this argument, then, the sense of responsibility and guilt experienced by OCD patients who suffer from aggressive, sexual or blasphemous obsessions may indeed be producing at least some of their distress, but this sense of responsibility and guilt may nonetheless be regarded as a "normal response" to their abnormal experience. (It might be argued here that neutralising is not such a response, but this point will be addressed presently.) The foregoing objection suggests, then, that the cognitive-behavioural account may place the cart before the horse in assigning the feelings of responsibility and guilt experienced by OCD patients with aggressive, sexual or blasphemous obsessions a primary role, and it is therefore perhaps best to suspend judgment as to whether these feelings may be assigned such a role. Nonetheless, Rachman (1993) makes a noteworthy point when he links his position here with the observation that OCD patients are "excessively conscientious and excessively correct" people (p. 151). This view of some OCD patients as people of "tender conscience" is widely held (Reed, 1985, pp. 54–5) and clearly might be used to predict that – consistent with the cognitive-behavioural account – these patients might be more sensitive than others to thoughts, images or impulses with, for example, sexual or aggressive themes. An alternative explanation would suggest that obsessions with these themes may result from the inability of these patients of tender conscience to express sexual or aggressive feelings (see Section 4.7.3 and Chapter 8).

Even if the cognitive-behavioural account were entirely wrong regarding the manner in which the distress of OCD patients with blasphemous, sexual or aggressive obsessions is produced, the possibility would still be left open that these patients might be helped if their feelings of responsibility and guilt were addressed by some form of cognitive therapy. Whether or not they could be so helped would remain an empirical question, and indeed one that has as yet received little attention (Jakes, 1989b). A possible source of confusion in this area may be a tendency to mistake *therapeutic technique* for *theory*; the cognitive-behavioural account of OCD thus tends to present as the *causes* of the disorder precisely those of its features on which cognitive therapists would wish to concentrate in their interventions.

It is significant that Rachman (1993) remarks that psychological fusion most notably occurs in cases of OCD involving blasphemous, sexual or aggressive obsessions – when one considers other types of OCD difficulties, problems arise that are quite independent of those considered so far and that place still greater obstacles before the cognitive-behavioural account. Consider, for example, a typical case where a patient fears that he may not have properly checked his gas taps or cleaned his hands and consequently carries out checking or cleaning compulsions. The putative process of appraisal in such cases as these, on the one hand, must be different from the process in those cases involving blasphemous, sexual or aggressive themes, on the other. Where these latter themes are involved, the appraisal, as discussed earlier, may involve the patient's feeling guilty merely for having had such a thought or impulse, and any compulsion he performs may consist of attempts to make amends for these bad thoughts (or impulses/images, etc.). Nothing of this kind takes place where the patient fears checking or cleaning tasks may need attention and he carries out checking or cleaning compulsions as a result. Here, there is no bad thought (impulse/image) – that is, no thought (impulse/image) about which the patient feels guilty merely for having experienced it. Salkovskis has argued that the cognitive-behavioural account may still be applied to such instances as this. Amending an earlier unsuccessful attempt to accommodate these cases (Salkovskis, 1985, p. 577; Jakes, 1989a, pp. 673–4), Salkovskis suggests (1989) that the appraisals in these cases issue from such beliefs as the following: "not neutralising" when an intrusion has occurred is equivalent to "seeking or wanting the harm involved in the intrusion to happen". Yet all this really claims is that these patients are very concerned about carrying out checking and cleaning tasks properly and would regard their own failure to prevent possible misfortunes by these means as reflecting very badly on themselves. This is to claim little that any account of OCD would wish to deny. It is clear that patients with checking or cleaning difficulties care profoundly as to the outcomes of their checking or cleaning tasks and would feel very guilty about any misfortune that occurred as a result of their not completing these tasks properly. To point out that this is so does not explain the difficulties of these patients, but rather only points out one of the things about these patients that stands in need of explanation. One may conclude that the cognitive-behavioural account, in its present form, is not offering a substantial analysis of OCD difficulties of this kind.

At this point, consider the suggestion, offered in the case of blasphemous, sexual or aggressive obsessions, that such obsessions are appraised by OCD patients as an imperative signal for action. This is clearly so for some of the patients who experience obsessions of this kind – that is, the obsessions of some of these patients do indeed provoke compulsive behaviours. But any account of the difficulties of these patients would have to acknowledge this. Once again, however, this is not an explanation, but rather what needs to be explained.

The situation is not the same regarding the claim, already discussed earlier, that guilt is usually produced by such obsessions. It is suggested by some that in many cases, contrary to what was argued earlier, guilt plays only a minor role, and other forms of distress – disgust at the content of the obsession, for example – are more important. The cognitive-behavioural approach, then, in emphasising the role played by guilt, is certainly not just stating what any account of OCD would accept in such cases as these. It is, rather, offering a distinctive account of the distress experienced by these kinds of OCD patients, albeit an explanation to which objections have already been raised.

A failure to go beyond what any account of OCD would accept is observed as regards some of the findings of Freeston et al. (1992), which were offered by these authors in support of the cognitive-behavioural account. Freeston et al. examined the cognitive intrusions of normal volunteers. When these subjects were asked, for example, "To what extent would you feel responsible if the thought content [that is, the content of their cognitive intrusions] were to happen?" those who had previously reported that they engaged in compulsive activities tended to say that they would feel responsible to a greater extent than those who did not report such activities. Yet, even if one can generalise from such a finding as this to OCD patients, doing so would, in itself, tell us little that is of importance to the explanation of the disorder. Any account would recognise the existence of an exaggerated sense of responsibility in some OCD patients and expect this to be associated with the performance of compulsive behaviour in such patients.

2.8.2 The genesis of OCD

What, then, of the suggestion that a combination of appraisals and compulsive behaviour *produces* OCD? Why should one suppose that abnormal obsessions develop from normal obsessions, doing so by means of the effect of this combination on normal obsessions? Salkovskis (1989, pp. 679–80) cites empirical evidence that is supposed to support this suggestion; however, at best the evidence fails to accomplish this, and some of it may actually contradict the cognitive-behavioural model (England and Dickerson, 1988; Jakes, 1989b). There are other difficulties. The cognitive-behavioural account notes the occurrence of normal obsessions or intrusive cognitions as "a universal human phenomena[sic]" (Salkovskis, 1989, p. 678) and takes this occurrence as given. Yet whatever the processes that are involved in producing normal obsessions may be, they evidently cannot be the appraisals and neutralising behaviour that – according to the cognitive-behavioural account – transform such obsessions into a clinical problem. Appraisals and neutralising behaviour are the responses of vulnerable individuals to the occurrence of intrusive cognitions and have no role in the production of such cognitions in the first place.

The position of the cognitive-behavioural account here lacks parsimony. The differences between normal and abnormal obsessions – the latter being more frequent and intense – are explained entirely in terms of the effects of appraisals and neutralising on normal obsessions, yet these processes play no part at all in accounting for the occurrence of normal obsessions. A more parsimonious account would clearly allow the processes that it supposed to produce normal obsessions also to have some role in producing abnormal obsessions, simply by being present to *a greater degree* in the case of abnormal obsessions than they are in the case of normal obsessions. The cognitive-behavioural account, in its present form, attempts to rule this out even as a possibility, while providing no grounds for attempting to do so.

The foregoing objection to the cognitive-behavioural account may be used in the form in which it has been presented for those cases where it was suggested that appraisals may have some role in producing the distress of OCD patients (that is, in cases of obsessions with blasphemous, aggressive and sexual themes). In cases involving such obsessions as fears that one's hands are dirty or gas taps are not switched off, the argument needs to be altered somewhat. It has already been argued that the cognitive-behavioural account, in its present form, fails to make any substantial contribution by postulating the appraisals that it suggests in such cases as these. It follows from this that the supposed appraisal in these cases cannot play the role suggested for it by the cognitive-behavioural account – to reiterate, the supposed appraisal here is part of what needs to be explained.

It could still be suggested that neutralising plays the role assigned to it by Salkovskis in creating the clinical problem in such cases as fears that one's hands are dirty, or gas taps are not switched off. However, one can point out that this suggestion lacks parsimony, just as it has been argued to do in those cases involving blasphemous, sexual or aggressive themes. If neutralising plays no part in producing normal obsessions that involve such themes as fears that one's gas taps are not switched off – and, because it is a response to normal obsessions, neutralising evidently can play no such part – why should one suppose that the differences between normal and abnormal obsessions may be explained in such cases entirely in terms of the effects of neutralising?

2.9   Summary

It has been argued that most of those aspects of the behavioural/learning account of OCD that have been considered here meet with substantial difficulties. This account is correct in suggesting that many obsessions and compulsions are provoked by environmental cues and that exposure to these cues causes many patients to experience discomfort. It has been argued, however, that Rachman and Hodgson's attempt to explain the repetitiveness of some compulsions from a behavioural point of view is implausible and that behavioural/learning theorists may have exaggerated the importance of discomfort reduction to the maintenance of compulsive behaviour. Discomfort reduction is not necessary to explain the maintenance of such behaviour, and some brief remarks have been offered concerning how one might provide a common explanation for the maintenance of both discomfort-reducing and discomfort-increasing compulsions.

The behavioural/learning approach encounters difficulties in explaining both the aetiology of OCD and the paradoxical failures of its feared stimuli to extinguish. Bersch argues that the concept of incubation fails to meet these difficulties, and it has been argued here that the preparedness hypothesis also fails to do so. The question of how good an account of the selectivity of the stimuli seen in OCD can be provided by evolutionary arguments in general and the preparedness hypothesis in particular will be offered later (see Sections 3.4 and 3.5).

It has been noted that the behavioural/learning account provides only one explanation of why exposure with response prevention is effective with OCD. Rachman's account of those obsessions that are not provoked by environmental cues has helped inspire a new approach to the treatment of such obsessions. The efficacy of this approach has as yet not been established, however, and it has been argued that Rachman's account of these kinds of obsession, in which the supposed similarities between obsessions and phobic objects are stressed, fails to explain the occurrence of such obsessions. Doubts have also been raised about the value of an alternative theoretical approach, suggested by Rachman, in which obsessions are seen as a sign of unprocessed emotion.

It has been argued that the cognitive-behavioural account provides no very compelling reason for supposing that the appraisals it presents in the case of some instances of OCD (those involving blasphemous, sexual or aggressive obsessions) are either the primary source of distress or the mechanism (in conjunction with neutralising behaviour) that converts normal obsessions into abnormal obsessions. The interesting connection between some aspects of the cognitive-behavioural account as applied to cases of this kind, and the observation that OCD patients are sometimes people of tender conscience, was noted. A possible alternative explanation of OCD's occurring in such people was briefly considered. It was argued that in other cases of OCD, the appraisals cited describe what needs to be explained, rather than provide an explanation. The cognitive-behavioural account, in making many of the same assumptions as the behavioural/learning approach, may also face some of the difficulties introduced here for that approach – for example, the cognitive-behavioural approach may, in its present form, share the inability of the behavioural/learning approach to explain the memory failures that accompany some such behaviour.

Other behavioural approaches to the treatment of OCD – especially the use of assertion training with some instances of the disorder (Emmelkamp and van der Heyden, 1980) – will be discussed later (see Section 4.7.3 and Chapter 8).

3 Accounts of OCD based upon personality theories derived from the work of Pavlov

3.1 Introduction

Numerous authors writing under the influence of Pavlov's (1928) seminal contribution have stressed the importance of individual differences in personality (or "temperament") to the explanation of OCD and other dysthymic disorders (for example, neurotic depression, phobias, etc.). Most notable among these authors is Eysenck, through whose work (e.g., 1952, 1979) this personality theory approach is linked to the behavioural/learning account of OCD and phobias (see Chapter 2). A brief outline of this approach, along with some points of general relevance to it, will be followed by more detailed discussions of two recent contributions from this school – those of Gray (1982) and Claridge (1985) – and, in particular, the accounts these authors offer of OCD.

3.2 Eysenck's account, and suggested modifications of it

As discussed in Section 2.1, Eysenck considers OCD and phobias to result from the operation of conditioning mechanisms. Consistent with this, he holds that those people who are most inclined to develop conditioned responses (argued to be those who tend toward neurotic introversion) are those in whom these disorders are most likely to be observed.

Gray (1970) suggests, among other modifications of Eysenck's account, that it may only be in settings involving signals of "frustrative non-reward" or punishment that neurotic introverts are more inclined to develop conditioned responses.

Gray (1979, 1982) also denies, as does (to some extent) Claridge (1985), that it is the hypothesised greater inclination among neurotic introverts to develop conditioned responses that explains most cases of OCD and phobias. The preparedness hypothesis is thus rejected by these authors – particularly in Gray's account – in favour of an explanation of most cases of OCD and phobias in terms of higher levels of innate fear among neurotic introverts.

3.3 OCD and neurotic introversion

Both Eysenck and Gray argue that it is neurotic introverts among whom OCD is most likely to be observed, and they would thus agree with Claridge (1985, pp. 72–3) when he states that patients with this disorder are "generally...introverted and highly neurotic on tests like the Eysenck questionnaires". This claim was not supported by the patients in the study reported by Jakes (1992, pp. 95–6). This study included groups of ten cleaners (OCD patients for whom cleaning compulsions were a major difficulty and who reported no checking compulsions of clinical severity), ten checkers (OCD patients for whom checking compulsions were a major difficulty), ten psychiatric controls (patients with various phobic difficulties), ten normals (who had no psychiatric history) and ten ex-patients (who had formerly been, but could no longer be, diagnosed as suffering from OCD). The scores of these groups on the Extraversion (E) scale of the Eysenck Personality Questionnaire (EPQ; Eysenck and Eysenck, 1975) were not as would have been predicted by this school of personality theorists – in particular, it was found that the scores of the checkers (mean = 12.7, sd = 5.7), psychiatric controls (mean = 9.2, sd = 5.1) and normals (mean = 12.3, sd = 6.4) were much higher than those of the cleaners (mean = 6.8, sd = 4.2). It was found that the scores of the ex-patients (mean = 8.3, sd = 3.7) were somewhat higher than those of the cleaners, but not as high as those of the other three groups (five of the ex-patients had formerly been cleaners, three had been checkers). The difference between the cleaners and checkers was statistically significant (p < 0.05), as was that between the cleaners and normals (p < 0.05). The difference between the psychiatric controls and cleaners fell short of significance. The checkers and psychiatric controls did not differ significantly from one another and neither of these groups was significantly different from the normals. There were no significant differences between the scores of the ex-patients and those of any of the other groups.

In this sample, then, neither checkers nor psychiatric controls confirm the prediction that low E scale scores will be recorded among patients suffering from dysthymic disorders; only the cleaners corresponded to this profile. The finding that among OCD patients it is checkers who do not confirm this prediction is especially surprising from the point of view of Gray's (1982) account (see Section 3.6). The prediction that ex-OCD patients would score low on this scale was also not confirmed, although there was a nonsignificant tendency for scores in this group to be lower than those of the normals.

As regards their Neuroticism (N) scale scores, the groups were more as would have been predicted by Eysenck's school of personality theorists. The cleaners (mean = 19.3, sd = 2.5), checkers (mean = 16.9, sd = 4.3) and psychiatric controls (mean = 16.5, sd = 5.2) all had high scores on this scale in contrast to the scores of the normals (mean = 6.5, sd = 5.2). The ex-patients (mean = 14.8, sd = 6.0) also scored much higher than the normals, although not quite as high as the other three groups. The differences between the cleaners, checkers, psychiatric controls and ex-patients on the one hand, and normals on the other, were all highly significant (p < .01). There were no other significant differences between the groups.

3.4 Preparedness and innate fear

It was argued earlier that the preparedness and incubation hypotheses are unable to deal with two difficulties that confront behavioural/learning accounts: the lack of evidence that the stimuli that elicit fear/discomfort in OCD and in phobias have been paired with aversive stimuli, and the failure of the stimuli that elicit fear/discomfort in OCD and in phobias to undergo extinction. Neither of these two difficulties arises with an account that retains the evolutionary argument of the preparedness hypothesis but abandons the role that the hypothesis assigns to conditioning mechanisms (thus also obviating the need for Eysenck's 1979 incubation hypothesis). Such an account, along with Gray's (1979, 1982) and (to a lesser extent) Claridge's (1985), would treat the fear/discomfort-eliciting cues involved in OCD and phobias as innate.

In support of his "innate fear" position, Gray (1982, pp. 429–34) argues that the findings from experiments conducted by Ohman and his co-workers, and presented by them in support of the preparedness hypothesis, are at least equally consistent with an innate-fear account. Gray further suggests (1979, 1982) that there is an observation that is consistent with the innate-fear account but which the preparedness hypothesis is unable to accommodate – namely, that the onset of some phobias (and, one might add, much OCD) tends to occur at certain ages. Gray suggests that the preparedness hypothesis, if it is to account for this observation, must suppose that conditioning experiences predominate at these ages, which is no more plausible, he argues, than the supposition that conditioning experiences tend to occur only in the presence of certain stimuli – and it was the implausibility of this latter suggestion that led to the introduction of the preparedness hypothesis in the first place.

Against Gray's objection concerning the ages of onset of some phobias, a defender of the preparedness hypothesis might argue that the preparedness of stimuli has its onset at certain ages, which is no less plausible than the same suggestion as regards innate fear, on which Gray's position is based. But, in order to explain why fear/discomfort will begin to be elicited by stimuli shortly after the onset of their preparedness, this defence of the preparedness hypothesis would also need to suggest that potential conditioning experiences are common. Against this suggestion, and in favour of Gray's objection, it has already been noted that potential conditioning experiences are *not* common. Given this, it therefore appears that Gray has indeed raised a further problem for the preparedness hypothesis.

Gray also argues that, consistent with his account of human fear, there is an abundance of evidence for the existence of innate fears of a wide variety of stimuli in a diversity of species, "including fear of snakes in monkeys never before exposed to them" (1982, pp. 434–5). Against this, Minneka (1986) has presented evidence that, she suggests, is more compatible with the fear of snakes among primates being prepared rather than innate.

3.5   Evolutionary accounts and OCD

As Gray notes, a great regularity has been reported regarding the kinds of obsessions and compulsions that are observed both within and between "widely differing places" (1982, p. 441). In both England (Rachman, 1978) and New Delhi

(Akhtar et al., 1975), the commonest obsessions concern dirt and contamination, the next most common in both places concern orderliness and aggression, followed by those that concern religion and sex. The most common compulsions reported in both England and India are also similar, involving cleaning, checking and tidying up. An attempt is made to explain some or all of this selectivity in exactly the same terms by both the preparedness and the innate-fear accounts – in terms, that is, of the supposed evolutionary advantage conferred by fear/discomfort concerning the items in question. But how good an explanation can be provided in these terms? This question is fundamental to both the innate-fear and the preparedness hypotheses.

Two preliminary points are worth noting. Firstly, all evolutionary arguments in this area tend to be of a highly speculative character, including those that are to be defended here. (De Silva, Rachman and Seigman's [1977, p.55] remark that "evolutionary arguments...are rather slippery and can be glibly made" is probably worth bearing in mind.) Secondly, it seems on the face of things paradoxical to attempt an explanation of the very disabling degree of fear/discomfort observed in OCD in terms of some supposed evolutionary advantage that this level of fear/discomfort has bestowed. A far milder degree of fear/discomfort concerning the things that trouble OCD patients, such as that reported by many normals (Rachman and de Silva, 1978), could perhaps be most plausibly argued to have survival value. If this is correct, an evolutionary explanation of OCD would have to be supplemented with some account of how the mechanisms that produce this optimum degree of fear/discomfort sometimes malfunction, resulting in clinical levels of distress. The force of the evolutionary argument appears to be weakened, but not entirely undermined, by this need for supplementary hypotheses.

So, how good an account of the selectivity of the stimuli and behaviour involved in OCD can be provided in evolutionary terms? De Silva (1988) suggests that the contents of most obsessions are indeed "highly prepared in the sense that they could be considered to be biologically relevant for humans in terms of their evolutionary significance" (p. 200). (For the purposes of the present discussion it is irrelevant whether this argument is couched in terms of the "preparedness" or "innateness" of fears.) De Silva supports his assertion by citing the findings of de Silva et al.'s (1977) investigation, but there are, as will be seen, difficulties regarding the manner in which that investigation classifies fears and behaviour as "highly prepared".

Before turning to that investigation, consider the general nature of evolutionary arguments in this area. If one wants to argue that a given fear or behaviour has been selected by evolution as innate or prepared, it is not sufficient to point out that the fear in question is likely to have existed since antiquity; it must also be shown that this fear or behaviour could not have been selected on rational grounds. That is, if it seems likely that "pretechnological man" (de Silva et al., 1977, p.56) would have shared with modern man a fear of X, this is not sufficient to argue that this fear is innate or prepared. It must also be shown that pretechnological man could not have been sufficiently knowledgeable to have appreciated a genuine danger posed by X. If such an appreciation can explain pretechnological man's fear of X, then it is not necessary to postulate some further mechanism, such as the preparedness or innateness of X as a feared object, to account for this. Thus, one should not be tempted to suggest that, for example, lions and tigers are innate or prepared fears for human beings, however confident one might be that a fear of these animals would have been shared by pretechnological man.

Consider, then, how one might argue that snakes or spiders are prepared – or innate-fear stimuli for human beings. The argument would be as follows: (1) Although many kinds of snakes and spiders have posed a threat to the survival of human beings (and other mammals) over countless years, this threat is not obvious, in the sense that it does not, for example, relate to such physical characteristics as the size or strength of spiders and snakes. (2) The acquisition by human beings (and other mammals) of innate or prepared fears regarding snakes and spiders would therefore be of value to survival by counteracting the absence of any "obvious" threat posed by the genuinely dangerous members of these species.

This argument does indeed appear to provide some reason for supposing the fear of snakes and spiders in human beings to have some evolutionary basis. It also makes possible an explanation of why fears of snakes and spiders are found in children too young to appreciate the genuine threat posed by some members of these species and (of more relevance to the present discussion) why people are scared of spiders and snakes that they know to be harmless. (In order to explain this fear of harmless spiders and snakes it is necessary to assume that the mechanism by which innate or prepared fears are acquired is not sufficiently subtle to distinguish between threatening and nonthreatening spiders and snakes.)

The investigation by de Silva et al. (1977) classifies as a "highly prepared behaviour" the "checking of fire hazards" and thus includes among such behaviour the very common OCD difficulty of checking light switches and plug sockets for fear that a fire might otherwise be caused. The problem with this classification should be evident from the foregoing discussion. It seems reasonable to suppose that a fear of fire hazards would indeed have been seen in pretechnological man, but this seems reasonable precisely because it is very likely that pretechnological man would have been able to appreciate, on rational grounds, the threat posed by such hazards – therefore, there would be no work here for prepared – or innate-fear mechanisms to do. Our reason for thinking that pretechnological man would probably have feared potential fire hazards is thus the same as our reason for thinking that this fear is not prepared or innate.

This is not to suggest, of course, that the OCD patient's checking of plugs and light switches is rational and is just a matter of the patient's recognising the genuine threat posed by potential fire hazards. This is clearly not so. The endless repetition of such checking, the patient's inability to remember earlier checks, his need to carry out some exact number of checks – none of these is merely a matter of the patient's recognition of genuine threat. But at best, evolutionary arguments seem likely to provide weak explanations of such maladaptive behaviour. This claim is consistent with what has been argued earlier – that evolutionary arguments are better at explaining why some stimuli are selected as aversive than they are at explaining very disabling degrees of fear, or indeed any other maladaptive behaviour, with respect to these stimuli. Explanations of such fears and behaviour, including the repetitive compulsions and failures of memory frequently observed in OCD patients with checking difficulties, must be sought in other terms.

As regards the question of why it is that plug sockets, light switches and door locks are frequently the items with which OCD checkers have most difficulty, a quite straightforward answer seems most probable: These are the items that most people usually have to check in the course of an average day. Items that people who are not OCD patients rarely check – for example, fuse boxes and electrical wiring – are more rarely problems for OCD patients. (Explanations couched in terms of the evolutionary significance of potential fire hazards are, of course, probably silent about this contrast between light switches and plug sockets on the one hand, and fuse boxes and electrical wiring on the other.) The selection of plug sockets, light switches and door locks as problems for OCD checkers is, therefore, simply a matter of these being the things that most of us need to check. It is no surprise at all, therefore, that people with checking difficulties most frequently have problems with these things. It must be emphasized that this explanation of *what* OCD patients usually check unfortunately tells us nothing at all about *why* these patients have checking difficulties. Explanations of this must be sought elsewhere.

Evolutionary arguments may be somewhat more plausible regarding other OCD difficulties. Gray argues that "the frequent choice of handwashing as the compulsive ritual" and the selection of dirt as "the commonest of obsessional preoccupations" reflect the fact that "natural selection may have favoured fear of dirt and its attendant grooming behaviour as much as fear of snakes or enclosed spaces". "Certainly", he suggests, "the danger to survival is no less great" (1982, p. 443).

Why, then, is this argument more plausible than that concerning fire hazards? This is because the danger that dirt would be argued to pose to survival is, like that posed by snakes and spiders in the earlier examples, not obvious. It is a relatively recent discovery that dirt may carry germs and disease, and pretechnological man would thus not have been sufficiently knowledgeable, in contrast to the case of fire hazards, to appreciate the threat posed.

A problem arises here. As pointed out earlier, the reason for supposing that pretechnological man would have feared potential fire hazards – namely, his being able on rational grounds to appreciate the threat such hazards pose – is also a reason for doubting that such hazards are prepared or innate fears. The situation as regards the aversiveness of dirt is precisely the reverse. As argued earlier, an innate or prepared aversion to dirt would have been of survival value to pretechnological man because he would not have been able to discern on rational grounds the threat that dirt posed to his survival. But this absence of rational grounds for pretechnological man's aversion to dirt also makes it far more difficult to be sure that he would have had any such aversion.

It seems to be difficult to produce very good evidence that species other than our own find dirt aversive. Thus, Gray himself adds the qualification of "obviously speculative" to his suggestion that there may be "an evolutionary continuity between the human use of soap and water and...[the] grooming behaviour [of animals]" (1982, p. 443).

Of greater interest would be evidence of OCD patients' being preoccupied with dirtiness and cleaning in societies (past or present) in which it was (or is) not known that dirt carries germs. (A milder aversion to dirt on the part of normals in such societies would similarly be of interest.) This would still not, of course, amount to conclusive evidence that an aversion to dirt has been "favoured by evolution". Social and religious pressures within such societies, for example, might be argued to account for the "selection" of these preoccupations by their OCD patients. But the existence of these pressures in such societies may not weaken the evolutionary argument very much – these pressures would themselves be argued to reflect the innate or prepared status of the aversion to dirt in human beings.

Evolutionary arguments seem likely to provide only weak explanations of the common occurrence in OCD of an array of other preoccupations and activities, such as the ordering of objects and "religious obsessions" (for example, blasphemous thoughts). Gray (1982, pp. 443–4) tries to explain both ordering and religious obsessions, as well as obsessions that are aggressive or sexual thoughts or impulses (see Section 3.6), as reflecting various activities on the part of a hypothesised "Behavioural Inhibition System". But, as is to be argued, substantial difficulties confront the account of OCD in terms of the functioning of this system.

3.6   Gray on OCD

3.6.1   *The Behavioural Inhibition System: an outline of Gray's account*

Gray (1982) presents his account of OCD in the context of his theory of anxiety. The central psychological concept of this theory is the Behavioural Inhibition System (BIS). Much of Gray's investigation consists of a search for "the neural structures that might subserve the functions" (p. 424) ascribed to that system. At this level, according to Gray, the activity of the septo-hippocampal system partially corresponds to the functioning of the BIS.

Gray distinguishes between (1) the "comparator or monitoring capacity ('just checking')" of the BIS (p. 425), in which it functions continuously but does not exercise direct control over behaviour, and (2) its functioning in those special conditions where it does exercise such control. The chief function of the BIS is performed in its comparator capacity, in that it monitors "ongoing behaviour, checking continuously that outcomes coincide with expectations" (p. 442). Incoming sensory information is scanned for "threatening or unexpected events" (p. 442). The special conditions in which direct control is exercised over behaviour are, in Gray's account, those where threatening or unexpected events are detected – those, that is, where a "mismatch" is detected between outcomes and expectations. In these conditions, according to Gray, the system interrupts ongoing motor programmes, checks whether alternative programmes lead to more satisfactory outcomes, and in addition may take control over exploratory and investigative behaviour (p. 425). Gray also describes the BIS as increasing "attention to environmental stimuli and [increasing the] level of arousal" (p. 424) when it takes control of behaviour.

The account of OCD offered by Gray against this theoretical background is presented via a critique of behavioural/learning explanations. Gray points out that such explanations, as has also been argued elsewhere (Section 2.6), fail to account for the occurrence of certain obsessions. He also suggests that a common explanation of the repetitiveness of obsessions and compulsions should be sought and that behavioural/learning accounts fail to make sense of the repetitiveness of either. It is the functioning of the BIS, according to Gray, that provides such an explanation. As discussed earlier, the chief function of this system is to scan incoming sensory information for threatening or unexpected events. Gray explains that this scan involves certain stimuli's being tagged as important and searched for with particular care. Were such a system to become hyperactive and thus "to tag too many stimuli as 'important' [and search] for them too persistently", what else would it produce, Gray asks (p. 442), but the repetitive thinking and behaviour that is symptomatic of OCD? Thus, the OCD patient is observed, Gray points out, "to scan his environment to an excessive degree for potential threats...much of this scan being carried out overtly, in the form of checking rituals" (p. 442). (It is perhaps unclear from Gray's account whether it is the patient's checking behaviour, or just his urges to carry out such behaviour, that Gray hypothesises to be under direct BIS control.) This scan for potential threat can, Gray furthermore suggests, "extend to internal repositories of information concerning such threats" (p. 442), so that the patient who is anxious about cutting himself "checks his memory to verify where he disposed of a razor blade, or wonders whether he saw a splinter of glass on a table" (p. 443).

Gray does not restrict his account to those symptoms that would usually be considered to involve the checking of the environment or internal repositories of information. For example, Gray suggests that handwashing "is at once an effective means of searching for dirt and a way to remove it"; the behaviour serves, that is, a checking as well as a cleaning function. The type of internal scan discussed earlier may also explain, Gray argues, the occurrence of impulses. The scanning of those systems that produce the behaviour that the patient is afraid to carry out may prime those systems to produce the behaviour in question, Gray suggests (p. 443), leading to the patient's experiencing impulses to perform that behaviour.

3.6.2 *OCD, anxiety and anxiolytic treatments*

There are two points that Gray stresses in applying his theory to anxiety disorders in man. Firstly, that the strengths of his account are "most apparent when it is applied to the obsessive-compulsive neurosis" (1982, p. 428), and secondly, that his theory has been derived from sources of data that are quite independent of that neurosis. These sources of data are "the results of purely behavioural experiments" with "the behavioural effects of the anti-anxiety drugs also [playing] an important part" (p. 424).

The second of Gray's points is especially important. According to Gray, the account of OCD that is provided by his theory might appear at first to be almost *too* good – it gives a "description [that] might seem too close to the phenomena to count as an explanation at all" (p. 442). It is the independence of the account's sources that ensures it an explanatory status and that makes its close fit with the phenomena of OCD the "most apparent" strength of the theory – an especially noteworthy strength, according to Gray, because, as compared with phobias, OCD presents "a much higher hurdle" (p. 439) for theories of anxiety, a hurdle that other laboratory-based accounts (that is, behavioural/learning accounts) have failed to clear.

A prediction that seems to follow from these two points stressed by Gray is that anti-anxiety drugs should be effective in reducing the symptoms of OCD. This prediction seems, indeed, to be crucial to the theory – the effects of these drugs have played an important part in the construction of the theory, and the most important strength of this theory, as applied to anxiety disorders in man, is considered by Gray to be the account it provides of OCD. Yet the prediction is at best highly contentious. Fineberg (1990) has suggested that OCD differs from anxiety disorders in several fundamental ways, including its failure to respond to "most conventional anxiolytic treatments", a claim with which Montgomery (1990) agrees.

Other contrasts emphasised by Fineberg (1990) are that, compared with anxiety disorders, OCD has a later age of onset and a different gender ratio (males and females being equally affected in the case of OCD, as against a female predominance in the case of anxiety disorders). Both Montgomery (1990) and Fineberg (1990) have suggested, on the basis of such contrasts between OCD and anxiety disorders, that the rationale for the current classification of OCD with these disorders is weak. It is of interest that doubts as to the status of OCD as an anxiety disorder have been independently raised on *phenomenological* grounds, by, for example, Reed (1985, 1991), Beech and Liddell (1974), and Rachman and Hodgson (1980). These doubts, then, raise another, albeit related, problem for Gray's account, which, in contrast to behavioural/learning approaches, seems to be committed to viewing anxiety as the major mood disturbance in OCD (see Section 2.1).

3.6.3 *BIS hyperactivity and checking behaviour*

Contrary to Gray's suggestion (1982, p. 442), it is not very clear that a hyperactive BIS would produce checking behaviour. Crucial to the present point is the distinction between the *monitoring* function of the BIS, in which the BIS does not exercise direct control over behaviour, and the functioning of the BIS that takes place in response to the detection of "threatening or unexpected" events and in which direct control over behaviour is exercised. One must suppose that the behavioural and cognitive symptoms that will result from the BIS's becoming hyperactive will be restricted to that behaviour and those thoughts that could be produced by the functions that the system performs when it takes control over behaviour. The monitoring by a hyperactive BIS would indeed involve, as Gray argues, too many stimuli's being tagged as important and being searched for too persistently. But this tagging and searching, it seems reasonable to infer from Gray's account of the functioning of the BIS, would not be reflected by the patient's overtly scanning his environment in the form of checking rituals, contrary to what Gray actually suggests (p. 442). No reason, that is, has been given for thinking that the monitoring function of a hyperactive BIS would exercise direct control over behaviour. Yet it is precisely the similarity between the monitoring function of the BIS and such scanning behaviour on the part of OCD patients that is stressed by Gray (p. 442) and that gives his account of OCD in terms of the functioning of the BIS its apparent plausibility. It seems, then, that Gray must either (a) explain why in OCD the monitoring function of the BIS begins to control behaviour directly or (b) instead explain OCD in terms of those functions the BIS is ordinarily hypothesised to perform when it takes control over behaviour.

3.6.4 *The BIS and Gray's dimensional approach*

As discussed in the foregoing section, Gray suggests that in its monitoring capacity the BIS does not exercise control over ongoing motor programmes, such control only being exercised under conditions of mismatch. It would seem, then, that the system is not involved in ordinary checking behaviour such as that performed by a careful person's locking the house at night. Such behaviour is rather, in the terms of Gray's theory, an ongoing motor programme. It follows that Gray's account implies a *qualitative* difference between checking that is symptomatic of OCD and normal checking behaviour – a qualitative difference in the sense that it implies that different brain mechanisms subsume normal checking and checking that is symptomatic of OCD. The extent to which this implication in itself counts as an objection to Gray's theory is perhaps unclear, although it is worth noting de Silva's (1988) suggestion that much "obsessive-compulsive symptomatology does not seem to be qualitatively different from what is usually regarded as normal" (p. 201). But it seems clear that the implication of a qualitative difference probably conflicts with Gray's own position, which is that, as regards anxiety disorders (OCD being included here among such disorders), a *dimensional* approach is most appropriate (p. 426). According to Gray there are, that is, "continuous distributions of behavioural propensities" as regards such disorders, with "those individuals who need psychiatric attention simply [being] located near the extreme pole of one or other of these dimensions" (p. 426).

Other difficulties for Gray's account as applied to OCD have been raised elsewhere. De Silva (1988) argues that the view of "cleaning rituals as checking-cum-cleaning behaviours" conflicts with "clinical observations" (p. 212). De Silva also argues that, contrary to Gray's suggestion, the evidence does not really favour a unitary explanation of both obsessions and compulsions. This argument may be reinforced by the suggestion (Section 1.3.4.5) that although there is no parallel to the repetitiveness of compulsions in the behaviour of phobic patients, the repetitiveness of some phobic thinking is indistinguishable from that of the obsessions experienced by some OCD patients. De Silva's objection may nonetheless be answered if it is only the *urges to perform* compulsive behaviours, rather than compulsive behaviours as such, that are being argued by Gray to be under direct BIS control. (It has been noted that Gray's account appears to be ambiguous on this distinction.) If it is only the urges to perform compulsive behaviours that are under direct BIS control, Gray's account can probably be reconciled with the contrasts between such behaviours and the obsessions on which de Silva's objection is based.

3.7   Claridge on OCD

3.7.1   *Anxiety in animals and man: Claridge's views on Gray*

Claridge denies that a complete account of OCD or phobias can be provided solely in terms of the individual differences in temperament that are associated with anxiety – that is, in terms of the differences that are central to the approach of Eysenck's school of personality theorists. Claridge therefore emphasises the necessity, as he sees it, also to include in any account of these disorders psychological processes that are unique to human beings, the physical instantiation of which, in contrast to the structures that are central to Gray's account, will be in humans' higher nervous system.

In suggesting this, Claridge takes himself to be rejecting Gray's claim that it is untenable to attempt any explanation of human anxiety in terms that are specific to human beings. Thus, Gray argues on the basis of the "precise similarity of the brain mechanisms responsible for anxiety in both rats and men" that "any attempt to explain human anxiety in terms that are specific to man (by recourse, say, to the vagaries of the Oedipus complex)" is "at once [ruled] out of court" (Gray 1982, quoted in Claridge, 1985, p. 72).

Claridge is correct to reject this claim. Even if Gray is right in asserting that the brain mechanisms that subsume the experience of anxiety in human beings and animals are largely the same, this assertion is quite compatible with the view that human beings and animals do not become anxious about the same things – and this view is the position common sense would take with regard to the present question. Thus, the relative complexity or abstract nature of some matters – being in debt or having a terminal illness, for example – means that only human beings can understand them and thus sometimes become anxious about them. It is reasonable, furthermore, to suppose that the capacity to understand such matters is unique to human beings, because humans are endowed with brain mechanisms that are peculiar to their species. But this supposition is entirely compatible with Gray's claim that the state of being anxious is itself mediated in human beings and animals by largely the same brain mechanisms. One must distinguish here between *that which* a person (or animal) is anxious about and the *anxiety* that is experienced by the person (or animal). (A possible source of confusion here is that one may describe as the "cause" of a person's anxiety both what the person is anxious about and the operation of those brain mechanisms that mediate the anxiety.) This is not to deny that it may be possible, at a sufficiently general level, to describe in exactly the same terms what both human beings and animals become anxious about, and Gray (for example, 1982), indeed, attempts to do precisely this when he places many of the stimuli that provoke anxiety in both human beings and animals under the common heading of "signals of punishment or frustrative non-reward". But this is entirely consistent with all of what has been said so far and, in particular, does not deny that some signals of punishment and nonreward may be unique to humans. Thus, it seems that the Oedipus complex, to take Gray's example, involves both signals of punishment (from the father) and nonreward (from the mother) – despite the complex's supposedly being such that if it were to exist, it would only be found in humans.

The fears observed in infrahuman species may nonetheless sometimes be used to help rule out those explanations that account for the fears reported by human beings and that are couched exclusively in terms specific to human beings. Thus, it is surely unparsimonious to attempt such a human-specific explanation of, for example, the fear of snakes, found in some people, given that this fear is also observed in some monkeys. The most plausible explanation of such a fear in people will be one couched in at least partly the same terms as those that can also be used to provide an explanation of this fear in monkeys. But the force of this argument, in contrast to that presented by Gray, is derived from the fact that in this argument it is not merely the brain mechanisms responsible for mediating anxiety, but the *feared object* as well, that is the same for both humans and animals.

3.7.2 OCD: Claridge's account

Drawing on the work of Beech and Liddell (1974) concerning the nature of the mood disturbance in OCD, as well as on the work of psychodynamic writers, Claridge argues that OCD may result when "emotionally reactive" individuals – by which he means those who are highly neurotic and introverted – are "brought up in family environments that happen to place undue emphasis on cleanliness, sexual repression and control of anger" (Claridge, 1985, p. 74). According to Claridge, this kind of upbringing may help to produce in such individuals the anxious guilt at sexual and aggressive feelings that produces much compulsive behaviour.

Claridge suggests that such anxious guilt may operate in conjunction with a characteristic cognitive style exhibited by people who are predisposed to OCD. Claridge draws on the experimental work conducted by Reed (1969a) in which, according to Claridge, obsessional subjects were shown to have "more narrowly defined concepts" than controls. By inference from this, Claridge suggests that obsessionals may also have "a more narrowly focused mode of *attending* to stimuli" (Claridge, 1985, p. 75, original emphasis), as evidenced by the preoccupation with minute detail often seen in OCD.

Although Claridge (1985, p. 72) evidently regards as peculiar to human beings the hypothesised individual differences in attentional style on which the cognitive aspects of his account are based, there is no obvious reason for supposing that such individual differences in attentional style could not occur in other species. (Indeed, could the anxious guilt that Claridge also hypothesises to be at work in OCD perhaps be more plausibly presented as peculiar to human beings?)

Of possible relevance to this point is Claridge's own observation that "there is an inextricable link between those mechanisms that have to do with the general arousal of the brain and the processes, in the higher nervous system, which control the breadth and narrowness of attention...[T]he more emotionally aroused the organism is", Claridge explains, "the more focused its attention becomes" (1985, p. 75). Claridge therefore suggests that the extreme emotional reactivity that he argues is exhibited by OCD sufferers *combines* with the cognitive style that he also believes to be characteristic of these patients and produces the minute attention to detail often featured in their difficulties.

Claridge also briefly notes (1985, p. 76) that there is some evidence that subjects with obsessional personalities tend to show an "overdominance of the left [cerebral] hemisphere", which, he suggests, "through its strong association with the control of language, could account for...[the] intellectualised, repressive stance on the world" of such personalities.

Claridge's suggestions may be challenged on a number of points. Thus, his discussion, like Reed's 1985 account, fails to make sense of the numerous types of OCD symptoms that fail to exhibit the characteristics stressed in Reed's analysis (see Section 6.6.1). The experimental evidence available is in any event at best equivocal as regards Reed's suggestion that OCD patients are characterised by the cognitive style described in his analysis, and furthermore,there is – contrary to both Claridge and Reed – arguably no evidence at all that this cognitive style plays any role in producing the suffering of OCD patients (see Chapter 6). Regarding the experimental work Claridge cites in connection with both the hypothesis of left hemispheric overdominance in obsessionals and Reed's account, Claridge assumes too close a link between the obsessional *personality* and OCD (Pollack, 1979, 1987).

Claridge's account nonetheless possesses at least two interesting features. Firstly, a number of authors, writing from a variety of perspectives, have suggested, consistent with Claridge's account, that the manner in which some OCD patients deal with their aggressive feelings may be important in explaining their symptoms (see Chapter 8 for further discussion). Secondly, as is argued elsewhere (see Section 6.3), accounts of OCD such as Reed's, which are based on the hypothesised cognitive style of patients with the disorder, encounter difficulties in explaining the motivation of OCD patients, suggesting that such accounts can at best provide only partial explanations of the disorder. Claridge's account may be regarded as an interesting, if not entirely successful, attempt to provide such an account with the supplement it requires.

3.8 Summary

Both Gray's account and Claridge's suggest that OCD patients should tend to be introverted, but evidence has been presented that contradicts this claim. Among OCD patients, according to the evidence quoted earlier, introversion appears to be exhibited more by those patients whose major difficulty is cleaning than it is by those whose major difficulty is checking. If this finding turns out to be replicable, it will require that both Gray's account and Claridge's be modified. This, of course, leaves open the possibility that the neuroticism of OCD patients may play a role in producing their symptoms, as writers such as Eysenck, Claridge and Gray suggest, and indeed it may even be, once again consistent with the views of Eysenck, Claridge and Gray, that in those OCD patients in whom both introversion and neuroticism occur, these two features combine to play a role in producing the symptoms observed. But even if all of this is accepted, it is clear that such temperamental characteristics as neuroticism and introversion cannot deliver a full account of the symptoms reported by OCD patients. As has already been noted, these temperamental characteristics are supposed to be exhibited not only by patients suffering from OCD but also by patients with other dysthymic disorders (see, for example, Claridge, 1985, Chapter 5), and so these characteristics could not begin to explain why, for example, one patient develops neurotic depression or a phobia but another develops OCD. Similarly, there appears to be a wide gulf between, on the one hand, the mere emotional reactivity that is supposed to characterise neurotic introverts and, on the other, the bizarre preoccupations, repetitive behaviour and failures of memory that are reported by many OCD patients.

It is this gulf that Gray's account attempts to bridge, whereas Claridge tries both to do this and to explain – in terms of individual differences in attentional style – why some patients develop OCD rather than phobias or depression. Both of these accounts, it has been argued, meet with difficulties. Gray's appears for a number of reasons not to provide a plausible explanation of the various OCD symptoms he discusses – including those that involve checking difficulties, the phenomena for which this account appeared at first to provide an especially elegant explanation. It has been noted that Claridge's account possesses a number of important strengths, but it relies too heavily on Reed's formulation of obsessional difficulties and thus encounters a number of the problems faced by that formulation.

Perhaps the most powerful argument considered in this discussion of personality theories derived from the work of Pavlov – and one that owes very little directly to those personality theories – is that it may be possible to explain the contents of some OCD symptoms (particularly those involving, as Gray suggests, cleaning behaviour and/or fears of dirt/contamination) in terms of the evolutionary advantage that such fears and behaviour can be hypothesised to have bestowed. It was noted, however, that the contents of various other OCD symptoms could not be explained in these terms. In those cases where evolutionary arguments do possess some force, it was suggested that, once again consistent with Gray's and some of Claridge's remarks, the most plausible mechanism through which such evolutionary pressures could exercise an influence may be innately acquired fears, rather than prepared fears.

4   Janet on OCD

4.1   Introduction

Janet's classic contribution to the literature on OCD (1903) has still not been translated into English. Fortunately, Pitman has provided a highly readable synopsis of Janet's work (1984) as well as an interesting review/commentary (1987a), which will be used as the basis of the discussion here. In his review/commentary, Pitman presents a summary of Janet's ideas in three segments, each of which will be considered in turn here; the points Pitman himself offers will be considered in the course of commenting on Janet's work. Havens (1966) also provides an interesting account of Janet's contribution, some points from which will be briefly discussed in what follows, as will some of Reed's (1985) comments on Janet.

4.2   Janet on the clinical stages of psychasthenic illness

Janet includes OCD, among other conditions, in the category he terms *psychasthenic illness*. He divides this category into three stages, these being, from the least to the most severe, *the psychasthenic state, forced agitations,* and *obsessions and compulsions.* According to Janet, patients develop the less severe stages of the illness before the more severe and, similarly, lose the more severe stages of the illness before they lose the less severe.

The first stage of the illness – the psychasthenic state – involves the patient's feeling that actions have been unsatisfactorily or incompletely performed. Incompleteness in "perceptions" is also present, consisting of such experiences as derealisation and depersonalisation. Indecision, amnesia, poor control of thoughts, and "emotional insufficiencies" (that is, an inability to experience emotions fully) are reported by patients. A number of "physiologic insufficiencies" are also present – for example, insomnia, sexual impotence and backache.

The second stage of the illness – forced agitations – includes "mental phenomena" (for example, rumination and repetition), "motor phenomena" (for example, tics and agitations) and "emotional phenomena" (for example, phobias and anxiety). The third and most advanced stage of the illness – obsessions and compulsions – usually involves forbidden thoughts or acts of a sacrilegious, violent or sexual nature.

4.3   Commentary on the clinical stages of psychasthenic illness

4.3.1   The psychasthenic state and compulsive personality disorder

Pitman notes that Janet has been presented as holding that all OCD patients have premorbid obsessional personalities. Pitman suggests that this is not quite accurate. He accepts that most of the elements in DSM-III's definition of compulsive personality disorder are included in Janet's account of the psychasthenic state and that in the majority of cases this state would be considered by Janet to have endured long enough to be classifiable as what would today be termed a personality disorder. But Janet also observes, Pitman points out, that in some cases the psychasthenic state may develop acutely, and thus in these cases it can probably not be classified as a personality disorder. It is also worth noting that Janet includes in the psychasthenic state much that appears to have nothing to do with the compulsive personality or compulsive personality disorder at all – for example, experiences of derealisation and depersonalisation.

4.3.2   Psychasthenia, OCD and other neurotic disorders

Pitman notes that among the forced agitations, Janet includes symptoms that would today be given quite separate diagnoses, such as agoraphobia, panic disorder, social phobia and generalised anxiety. He suggests that Janet's inclusion of all of these disorders under the common rubric of forced agitations is supported by modern evidence of the co-morbidity of these disorders with one another and with OCD (Pitman, 1987a, p. 228). This stress on the similarities between OCD and the disorders with which it tends to be co-morbid is an interesting similarity between Janet's theorising and that of the Pavlovian personality theorists (see Chapter 3).

Pitman misrepresents Janet's position in suggesting that symptoms that would today be diagnosed as OCD appear only in the third and most severe stage of psychasthenic illness and that it is, therefore, surely unfortunate that only the symptoms seen in this stage are termed "obsessions and compulsions". Thus, in his review/commentary, Pitman gives as examples of forced agitations the following: symptoms that involve checking, repetition, and preoccupations with order and symmetry; a case involving "touching the pants to ward off the idea of a having been brushed by a rabid dog" (Pitman, 1987a, p. 227); and a case of "a knife phobia [*sic*] [that arises] out of an obsession with the act of homicide"(p. 227). It seems likely that these symptoms would all be diagnosable as OCD, and many similar examples are provided in Pitman's synopsis of Janet's work. Indeed, it is surely possible that some of the examples that Pitman provides of the symptoms seen in the psychasthenic state – for example, feelings that actions have not been performed well or completely – could in some cases be symptomatic of OCD. This is particularly so given the point already noted, which Pitman himself makes, that such features are in some cases not classifiable as compulsive personality traits because of their acute onset.

Pitman seems, therefore, to be similarly in error when he reviews as crucial to Janet's position the modern evidence concerning the question of whether or not patients report symptoms of OCD only after they have begun to exhibit disorders such as anxiety-depression, phobias and generalised anxiety disorder. (Pitman concludes that the modern evidence is equivocal on this point, although "more consistent [with what Pitman takes Janet's position to be] than contradictory" [Pitman, 1987a, p. 228].) Janet would appear to be committed, at most, to the claim that only *some kinds* of OCD – those involving thoughts of a sacrilegious, violent or sexual nature – should occur only after the appearance of (1) the other disorders that Pitman discusses as parts of the second stage of psychasthenic illness and (2) the kinds of OCD that, contrary to Pitman's interpretation, Janet evidently included in the second stage, and even in the first stages, of psychasthenic illness. It also seems, from Pitman's account of Janet's work, that not only instances of what today would be diagnosed as OCD are included in the third stage of psychasthenic illness. Thus, one example provided in Pitman's review of this stage of the illness involves "the belief that one is fat when one is actually thin" leading to "bizarre dieting with weight loss" (although see the discussion of Haven's work and "hysterical anorexy" in Section 4.7.1).

4.3.3 Psychasthenia, OCD and anxiety

Pitman stresses that Janet rejects anxiety-centred explanations of OCD, preferring an account in terms of the lowering of psychological tension, as will be discussed presently. Pitman suggests that within Gray's (1982) broader neuropsychological theory of anxiety (see Section 3.6) it may be possible to explain a number of the observations that, according to Janet, anxiety-centred accounts are unable to handle.

4.4 Janet on the hierarchy of psychological phenomena and psychological tension

Noting that not all psychological operations are equally impaired among psychasthenics, Janet constructs a hierarchy of such operations. Those operations that are at the top of this hierarchy are impaired in psychasthenic illness, those that are lower down are not. The highest level of the hierarchy is termed the *reality function* or the *function of the real* by Janet (Havens, 1966). It is difficult to state in just a few words what Janet means by this. Pitman says

> The highest level of the hierarchy is the reality function. This includes real actions that require high effort such as social adjustment and adaption to novel circumstances. Alongside real actions are real perceptions, including memories pertinent to

the real situation at hand, but not irrelevant ones. Also included are emotions adapted to present reality, especially happy emotions. Psychasthenics encounter numerous difficulties in dealing with real situations. They are rendered impotent by their shyness and have difficulty expressing even gratitude or tenderness...Novel social challenges are the most difficult for psychasthenics. (Pitman 1987a, p. 229)

Below the reality function in the hierarchy are "disinterested mental activities". As an example of these, Janet mentions the giving of advice to others, which, he suggests, psychasthenics often have little trouble with, despite being unable to make their own decisions (decision making being included at the reality-function level by Janet). Lower still in the hierarchy are thought processes having little to do with present reality – for example, imagination and abstract reasoning. Lower still are "non-specific emotional-viscerosomatic discharges typified by anxiety" (Pitman, 1987a, p. 229). Nonspecific motor agitation and tics occupy the lowest level.

Janet suggests that "two essential features characterise the highest level of the hierarchy: unification of novel mental synthesis and the richness of conscious elements that take part in it" (Pitman, 1987a, p. 229). According to Janet, it is a diminution in the capacity for "novel mental synthesis" that explains the psychasthenic's difficulties with volition and attention, and a "loss of the richness of conscious elements" that produces the experiences of depersonalisation and derealisation. The combination of these two essential features constitutes the characteristic Janet terms *psychological tension*, which he believes corresponds to "some physiologic tension" in the central nervous system. The amount of psychological tension possessed by an individual determines the highest point in Janet's hierarchy at which that individual can function. Janet suggests that psychological tension is lowered in the psychasthenic, and it is this lowering of tension that makes the completion of higher level operations impossible for him.

The inability to complete high-level operations leads to the appearance of phenomena such as agitations, tics and anxiety, because (on Pitman's account of Janet) the mental energy that would otherwise be used in the higher operations is diverted into psychological operations that are lower down in Janet's hierarchy. The forced agitations in psychasthenia are hypothesised to arise when the patient wishes to perform some high-level activity, such as initiating an action or making a decision.

4.5   Commentary on the hierarchy of psychological phenomena, and psychological tension

4.5.1 *Psychological tension*

Pitman makes an important point when he says that Janet's theory of psychological tension appears to rest upon a circular argument. We seem to be told by Janet that the reality function is impaired in psychasthenia because these patients have lowered psychological tension, but the reason Janet gives us for supposing the reality function to involve high psychological tension is that it is impaired in psychasthenia. Pitman's charge of circularity against Janet might be answered if the theory of psychological tension were applicable to conditions other than psychasthenia – indeed, as Pitman points out, one is entitled to expect the theory to be applicable to other conditions, given that it is supposed to reflect "a basic organisation of the central nervous system" (Pitman, 1987a, p. 230). But on the contrary, as Pitman again correctly observes (1987a, p. 230), the theory appears to lack such a wider applicability. Pitman points out that mentally handicapped people, for example, often have less difficulty with interpersonal relationships than with abstract reasoning, although it is interpersonal relationships that stand higher in Janet's hierarchy. Pitman also suggests that Janet's speculations that "some physiologic tension" in the central nervous system corresponds to the observed level of "psychological tension" would not be taken seriously by modern neuroscientists. Reed (1985), however, offers a quite different account of Janet's notion of psychological tension (see Section 4.5.4).

4.5.2 *The reality function*

There may be difficulties for Janet's suggestion that all the functions, and only those functions, that are included at the highest level of his hierarchy of psychological phenomena can be characterised as being involved in the negotiation of reality (see Section 4.4). The claim that *some* level-one functions may be contrasted with *some* lower-level functions in involving the negotiation of reality seems reasonable (despite Janet's unusual choice of terminology). For example, it probably is plausible to claim, as Janet does, that adjusting to novel social circumstances (a level-one activity) can be contrasted in these terms with abstract reasoning and introspection (level-three activities). But in what way are the sleeping difficulties of psychasthenics, for example, supposed to reflect a failure of the reality function? Havens (1966, p. 394) informs us that Janet regards such difficulties as reflecting a "failure of the act of sleeping". Yet even if one were to make the (substantial) concession that falling asleep is an act, this takes us no nearer an understanding of how the performance of this act involves the negotiation of reality. Nor, arguably, is it clear how the giving of advice to others (a level-two activity) involves less interaction with reality than does social adjustment (a level-one activity).

It is surely also implausible to suppose that *all* OCD patients exhibit *all* of the features included in Janet's psychasthenic profile. Thus, the difficulties of psychasthenics "in dealing with real situations" leads, Janet suggests, to their being "rendered impotent by their shyness." According to Janet, these patients "find on the stairway the word that needed to be said in the parlour" (Pitman, 1987a, p. 229). Janet also suggests that "if there is anything that [psychasthenics] find more painful than a decision, it is a fight" (Pitman, 1987a, p. 230). Memorable though these phrases are, one is however struck by how much these patients *differ* from one another with respect to such characteristics as their degree of shyness and timidity. Similarly, as discussed in Section 3.3, OCD patients' scores were found to vary considerably on some of the dimensions of personality studied by theorists working under Pavlov's influence (for example, Eysenck, 1979; Claridge, 1985; and Gray, 1982). Lewis also remarks that not all obsessional personalities are timid. Although some certainly are, being "vacillating, uncertain of [themselves and] submissive", others are by contrast "obstinate...[and] irritable" (Lewis, 1936, p. 328). Indeed, Janet himself remarks that psychasthenics may tend toward "authoritarianism" as well as "subordination" (Pitman, 1987a, p. 227).

Janet regards the activities that he places at level two in his hierarchy (such as giving advice to others) as intact in psychasthenia, and it is therefore evident that he thinks of only the highest level of his hierarchy as impaired in the illness. It is this selective impairment that Janet uses to justify his placing the activities that he supposes to be exercises of the "function of the real" at the top of his hierarchy, and it is therefore unclear, at least from Pitman's account of his work, on what basis Janet organises into levels the other psychological operations he discusses.

4.5.3 Psychasthenic illness and Janet's hierarchy

Janet makes no suggestion that the last stage of psychasthenic illness involves activities that are lower in his hierarchy of psychological phenomena than the activities involved in the first and second stages of the illness. Thus, Janet appears to hold that tics and other motor agitations (both included in stage two) occupy the very lowest level of his hierarchy; the obsessions and compulsions of stage three, understood as including thoughts of an aversive nature for the patient, can evidently not be included at this level and must therefore appear higher, perhaps most plausibly at level three. The last stage of the illness thus seems to be, if anything, characterised by activity that is *higher* in Janet's hierarchy than much of that seen in the first and second stages.

4.5.4 Displacement activity

Janet's suggestion that forced agitations result from the diversion of energy intended for other acts was, Pitman argues, a remarkable anticipation of the ethologic concept of *displacement activities*. Such activities "are currently considered a possible animal model of human compulsive behaviours", Pitman notes (1987a, p. 230), adding that these activities "typically occur in conflict situations". Pitman gives an example of displacement activity involving the stickleback fish, which has been observed to engage in nest-building activity while in the midst of a border dispute with a rival. This nesting behaviour is hypothesised to result from a conflict (in the stickleback exhibiting this behaviour) between the inclination to fight and the inclination to flight. Pitman stresses that this displacement behaviour is *out of context,* in that it is not attributable to either competing inclination (thus, neither fight nor flight behaviour would be out of context in this sense).

It is at this point that Pitman finds an element missing in Janet's psychological formulation. Janet fails, in Pitman's view, to recognise "the role played by intrapsychic conflict" in OCD (Pitman, 1987a, p. 228). Pitman argues elsewhere (1987a) that most cases of OCD can be seen as displacement arising from intrapsychic conflict over the expression of, for example, aggression and sexuality. Pitman thus suggests that OCD usually occurs because patients are motivated to act in ways they find unacceptable; this produces conflict that in turn gives rise to OCD and, in particular, to compulsive behaviours – such behaviours being classified by Pitman as displacement activities.

Pitman points out that Janet, by contrast, sees conflict and dissatisfaction as secondary – a *result* of volitional difficulties, not the *cause* of them. The picture of Janet's account that thus emerges here is one that provides half of the conflict/displacement model to which Pitman subscribes. Janet is presented as acknowledging the importance of displacement mechanisms but failing to provide any successful account of why they operate and, in particular, not recognising the role played by intrapsychic conflict.

A close reading of Pitman's own synopsis (1984) of Janet's work suggests that this picture overstates the similarities between Janet's work and Pitman's conflict/displacement model. It seems clear that Janet considers *some* of the symptoms of psychasthenic illness to arise by means of displacement mechanisms as described by Pitman. Thus, Janet talks of the necessity "to introduce...the concept of the diversion of mental energy, occurring when the primary avenue is blocked" and stresses that "various inferior phenomena...may substitute for one another in forced agitations, as if excitement had to be discharged somehow" (Pitman, 1984, p. 307).

But not all symptoms of the illness, nor even all forced agitations, are explained in terms of diverted energy by Janet. For example, he says that "the mania of repetition arises from the feeling of discontent with the way an action was previously performed, as does the mania of going back (checking)" (Pitman, 1984, p. 295). It is important to note again here that it is *only* those actions the performance of which involves the reality function that are affected by such feelings of discontent in psychasthenic illness. Thus, it would seem that the repetition and checking seen in symptoms such as those referred to in the foregoing quote are of *some action, the successful performance of which would place it at the highest level of Janet's hierarchy*, but which the patient is unable to perform successfully, in the sense that he cannot experience any satisfaction about the manner in which it has been carried out. This is, of course, entirely consistent with Janet's claim that the successful performance of these actions – meaning their being performed in the absence of feelings of discontent – is unavailable to psychasthenic patients. But this account seems to be clearly distinguishable from one based upon displacement mechanisms, in which checking and repetition result from the energy diverted from some *entirely different* act the patient has been unable to perform because of a conflict. Similarly, in cases of the type to which Janet refers in the quotation about manias of checking and repetition, there is no question of the patient's wishing to perform some action that he also regards as unacceptable. And nor is there, therefore, any suggestion that the conflict created by the wish to perform such an act is what makes acts of the type in question impossible for the patient to perform and that the resulting repetition and checking, as required by Pitman's conflict/displacement model, are of some *entirely different* and out of context behaviour. The checking and repetition in the type of cases discussed by Janet are of the very action the successful performance of which is unavailable to the patient. This action is thus not of a forbidden nature for the patient – it is not, that is, an action he would try not to carry out (his repetition and checking *are* his attempts to carry it out) – and the patient's checking and repetition are thus not of an action that is out of context in Pitman's sense.

Reed's 1985 account of Janet's work may be more consistent with these observations (also see Section 6.14). Reed (p. 78), in contrast to Pitman, sees Janet's notion of psychological tension as being a major advance in the understanding of OCD. Reed believes the notion to be widely misunderstood, Janet using it, Reed argues (p. 76), to mean *input integration* or *schematization*. Reed thus believes there to be a close connection between Janet's account and his own (see Section 6.1), in which the central problem in obsessionality is argued to be a "failure in spontaneous categorizing and integration" (p. 220). Reed regards some compulsive checking and repetition, for example, as resulting from the OCD patient's failure to categorize tasks as having been done properly or sufficiently, this in turn having resulted from the patient's inability to treat as irrelevant to this categorization trivial details concerning the exact manner in which tasks have been performed. The patient, in Reed's terms, is unable spontaneously to categorize (or integrate) the task, and this (according to Reed) is what Janet is also claiming when he hypothesises that psychological tension is lowered in psychasthenia.

Whether or not this is plausible as an interpretation of the notion of psychological tension, it is certainly more consistent with Janet's remarks concerning the nature of checking and repetition than is Pitman's displacement interpretation. The checking and repetition – on Reed's interpretation and required by Janet's remarks – will be of the very action that the patient's lowered psychological tension has rendered him unable to perform to his own satisfaction.

Some of Janet's remarks thus appear to provide support for Reed's interpretation of his work whereas others, as noted earlier, support the interpretation offered by Pitman. It seems, then, that neither interpretation can provide a full account of Janet's ideas and that some combination of these interpretations may come closer to a full account than either can alone. It is of some interest to note that, despite their contrasting accounts of Janet, both Pitman (1987a) and Reed (1985) believe there to be connections between Janet's work and cybernetic theory (see Section 3.5).

4.5.5 Conflict and OCD

Pitman seems a little too ready to criticise Janet for supposedly underplaying the role of conflict in OCD. Pitman's position on this point is very like that of

Havens (1966), both of them arguing, on the basis of the symptom contents of some OCD patients, that intrapsychic conflict over such matters as aggression and sex is involved. Havens, for example, presents the case (discussed by Janet) of psychasthenics who, tormented by the thought that they do not fully love their fiances, strive hard to do so and, as a result of these strivings – or so Janet argues – end up detesting them. (Let us assume here that the detestation toward their fiances would sometimes take the form of *obsessions* experienced by these patients, thus making some of these cases instances of OCD.) This account, that presents the experienced detestation as secondary to the inability to love, may be contrasted with what Havens suggests "the contemporary mind immediately grasps" (p. 392) – by which he means what would be suggested by a psychodynamic approach to such a problem, wherein the detestation reported would be presented as primary, and as having caused (when the detestation was still unacknowledged by the patient) the inability to love. Pitman similarly remarks (1987, p. 228) that "the modern reader with any psychodynamic leaning" cannot fail to spot this "error" in Janet's formulation of numerous cases. Havens, noting that Janet's patients are "again and again" reported as being horrified by their symptom content, thinks it remarkable that Janet did not move toward a "conception of mental illness as conflict" (Havens, 1966, p. 397).

Yet it is surely not *obvious* that the account Janet offers is for all cases inferior to the conflict-based one Pitman and Havens favour. Is it clearly the case, for example, that the detestation featured in Janet's example could not have arisen in the manner he postulates? Janet is surely not just clearly wrong here. On the face of things, that is, it seems that it may be possible to explain some aggressive symptom contents as secondary to the patient's frustration at his or her doubts and inability to feel or act.

Pitman also discusses his conflict/displacement account of OCD while presenting a cybernetic model of the disorder. Some comments on his discussion are offered in Section 4.9.3.3; also see Chapter 5, Section 7.6, and Chapter 8 for further remarks on conflict-based accounts of OCD.

4.5.6 The physiological basis of displacement

It is worth noting that Pitman is too optimistic about accepting Janet's "diversion of mental energy" or "displacement" explanation of (some) forced agitations while rejecting Janet's speculations regarding the physiological basis of this hypothesised process – the interdependence of the psychological and physiological levels of Janet's theorising is greater than Pitman evidently supposes. This is because it is more difficult to characterise adequately the notion of a displacement activity when using it, as does Pitman (1987a, 1987b), in the context of a psychological theory that makes no claim about the possible physical bases of the phenomena with which the theory deals. An account that suggests that a given conflict/distress is *displaced* in an activity must be distinguishable from accounts of that activity that instead argue, for example, that the activity provides *distraction* from that conflict/distress (or even, in some cases, relief from it via muscle relaxation). The observation that some compulsive behaviour always arises in the context of, and leads to a reduction in, conflict/distress (for example, anger the patient is unable to express) would thus not in itself be strong support for a displacement account of that compulsive behaviour. This observation would be equally consistent with the distraction (or even, in some cases, the muscle-relaxation) hypothesis.

Because Janet's displacement-activity account claims that there is some physiological displacement corresponding to the observed psychological displacement, it can be distinguished from these alternative hypotheses by virtue of its making this claim. These alternatives, in contrast to such a displacement account, do not seem to imply that it should be possible to observe the passage of activity from the CNS mechanisms that mediate the patient's experience of his conflict/distress to those CNS mechanisms that mediate the performance of his displacement activity. If, therefore, Janet's speculations as to physiological processes are, as Pitman suggests, implausible, then Janet's hypothesis that psychological displacement is taking place must also be weakened, contrary to Pitman's position.

4.6   Janet on diagnostic and treatment issues

Janet observes that "dissociative and conversion disorders" (Pitman, 1987a, p. 228), which he classifies as hysterical illnesses – his other major category of neuroses – are rarely co-morbid with those symptoms seen in psychasthenic illness. Janet draws a number of distinctions between hysterical and psychasthenic illness (and between the people who suffer from these two illnesses). For example, the pathological ideas of the hysteric are, according to Janet, readily translated into action, perception and belief, in contrast to the pathological ideas of the psychasthenic, and whereas hysterics are usually readily hypnotizable, psychasthenics are usually not. Havens (1966, p. 393) points out that Janet regards hysterics and psychasthenics as being distinguishable with respect to *the extent to which* they are able to "hold their ideas in full consciousness". Thus, whereas the hysteric exhibits a more complete dissociation, the psychasthenic experiences only a "partial dissociation" of his ideas (p. 393).

Heredity, according to Janet, plays an important but "not a tightly determining" role in psychasthenia (Pitman, 1987a, p. 231), and Janet suggests that the interbreeding of families with vulnerability to the illness should be avoided. Janet suggests that in individuals formerly in good psychological health, the illness may occasionally be produced by various stressors, but it is more usually a "longlasting constitutional condition" (Pitman, 1987a, p. 230) that is found in people who have always been of timid character and is exacerbated by precipitants such as losses, examinations and marriage. Psychasthenia is, Janet suggests, three times more common in women than men. The most common outcome of the illness, according to Janet, is a "relative recovery", usually before the age of

40 (Pitman, 1987a, p. 231). He notes that a minority of psychasthenics develop melancholia or paranoia.

The prevention of the disorder is most readily achieved, Janet suggests, by encouraging predisposed children to "confront reality" (Pitman, 1987a, p. 231) – the physical (for example, practical activity and even fights) should be encouraged over the intellectual for such children. The treatment of psychasthenia, according to Janet, should take the form of encouraging the patient not to doubt, and "to devote himself to a task and then stick it out". He believes that the patient should be "pushed in the direction that he really wants to go but cannot quite find it in himself to" (Pitman, 1987a, p. 231).

4.7   Commentary on diagnostic and treatment issues

4.7.1 *Hysterical and psychasthenic illness*

The theorising of some Pavlovian personality theorists (for example, Claridge, 1985) is once again brought to mind by Janet's distinction between, on the one hand, dissociative and conversion disorders and, on the other, OCD and the disorders with which it tends to be co-morbid. Janet's suggestion that action, perception and belief are not affected in psychasthenic illness is implausible, although his claim that hysterical illness and psychasthenic illness involve different degrees of dissociation is intriguing. This claim may be open to numerous interpretations, but each of these meets with difficulties. For example, in discussing the partial dissociation of psychasthenics, Havens (1966, p. 393) notes Janet's observation that at one moment the patient has full possession of his thoughts – he knows at that moment that he has not, for example, committed some crime – but then "the certainty diminishes and the ruminative doubting [i.e., as to whether he has committed the crime] resumes". But not all of the symptoms seen in OCD (and still fewer of those seen in psychasthenia) involve the doubting and uncertainty being used to justify reference to partial dissociation (see Section 1.3.4). Perhaps instead, then, the *insight* exhibited by psychasthenics as regards their pathological ideas should be used to characterise their disorder as involving only a partial dissociation of ideas. Partial dissociation would on this interpretation refer to the psychasthenic's *attitude toward* his symptoms – his agreeing with others about their morbid nature – instead of to doubts that are themselves *part of* the psychasthenic's symptoms (as in Janet's suggestion). And the contrast, on this interpretation, would therefore be between the psychasthenic's insight into his pathological ideas and the absence of insight that is observed during – and after – the occurrence of such hysterical symptoms as fugue states and somnambulisms. In reply to this, however, one must note that insight is not seen in all cases of OCD (Section 1.2.6; Stern and Cobb, 1978; Walker, 1973; and Jakes, 1992, Chapter 2), so this feature is also unable to support Janet's contrast of psychasthenic and hysterical illnesses in terms of the degree of dissociation involved.

This contrast is perhaps most plausibly defended in terms of another of Janet's remarks: Whereas "the hysteric appears not to know what troubles her...[the psychasthenic] knows perfectly well what torments him" (Havens, 1966, p. 392). The psychasthenic, that is, is more aware of what troubles him in that he does not exhibit amnesia with respect to his symptoms, in contrast to the amnesia concerning their symptoms that is exhibited by patients suffering from fugue states and somnambulisms (see Havens, 1966). But, against this position, it might be argued that not all patients suffering from hysterical symptoms are amnesic regarding them – the amnesia exhibited by patients suffering from fugue states and somnabulisms is not seen in all cases of hysterical illness. If this claim is correct, a clear contrast between psychasthenic and hysterical illnesses has still not been drawn.

This raises the question of which symptoms Janet classifies as psychasthenic and which as hysterical. There appears to be some dispute as to this question. According to Pitman (1987a, p. 228), Janet considers anorexia nervosa "to be a form of obsessive-compulsive behaviour" and thus a symptom of psychasthenic illness. Havens (1966), however, suggests that anorexia nervosa – termed by Janet *hysterical anorexy* – is classified by Janet as a hysterical disorder. It seems that anorexic patients could no more be described as amnesic with respect to their symptoms than could psychasthenic patients and that if Havens is correct as regards Janet's classification of anorexia nervosa, a clear distinction has yet to be provided between those symptoms Janet regards as hysterical and those he regards as psychasthenic based on the degree of dissociation their sufferers exhibit. It could at most be claimed that only *some* hysterical symptoms can be contrasted with the symptoms seen in psychasthenia in terms of degree of dissociation.

4.7.2 *Empirical evidence relevant to Janet's position*

Pitman suggests that Janet's comments on the role of heredity in psychasthenia agree with current thinking (also see Section 1.1) and that Janet is also correct in claiming that although most patients eventually improve, a small percentage develop signs of psychosis. Pitman takes issue with Janet's claim of a much higher incidence of psychasthenia in women compared to men. Pitman's objection, however, is based on the modern evidence concerning the gender ratio for OCD, and so Janet's inclusion in psychasthenic illness of phobic and other anxiety disorders in which there is, in contrast to OCD, a large female predominance (Fineberg, 1990) suggests Pitman's criticism to be unfair.

4.7.3 *Janet and behaviour therapy*

Pitman claims that the treatment recommendations of behaviour therapists were anticipated by the interventions suggested by Janet. Thus, Janet's prescription that children who are predisposed to psychasthenia should be encouraged to confront danger anticipated, according to Pitman, the "principle of direct therapeutic exposure," and Janet's prescription that psychasthenic patients should be prevented from doubting and encouraged to persevere with tasks, anticipated the behavioural technique of response prevention.

This appears to be an overstatement of the similarities between Janet's treatment recommendations and these behavioural interventions. The crucial ingredient of exposure and response prevention is that the patient is encouraged to confront *the stimuli and tasks that feature in his symptoms*, and is discouraged from carrying out the compulsive behaviour he usually performs *with respect to those stimuli and tasks* (see Section 8.4.3). This emphasis upon the patient's confronting those stimuli and that behaviour that feature in his symptoms is evidently absent from Janet's suggestion that predisposed children and patients merely be encouraged to take risks and to persevere with tasks. Indeed, Janet's position is that "because obsessions are symbolic expressions of an underlying state, treatment must be directed not at the symbol but at the state itself" (Pitman, 1987a, p. 231). This would, if anything, appear to be an anti-exposure position.

There may be other behavioural approaches to therapy that have more in common with Janet's recommendations. Emmelkamp and van der Heyden (1980) note, like Janet, the timidity of some OCD patients and attempt to use this observation both to help make sense of, and to treat, some kinds of OCD symptoms. Thus, Emmelkamp and van der Heyden suggest that "harming obsessions" – obsessions that feature the theme of hurting other people or oneself – result from unexpressed aggressive feelings, which in turn have resulted from the inappropriately unassertive behaviour of those patients who report such obsessions. Thus, Emmelkamp and van der Heyden note that patients with such obsessions, like the patients discussed by Janet, are inclined to be unassertive and that, at least in some cases, the most powerful precipitants of such obsessions are situations that require these patients to act assertively. One such situation, which Emmelkamp and van der Heyden give as an example, is that of being criticised unfairly by someone, which in the case of one patient they treated gave rise to obsessional thoughts about harming the person by whom the patient had been criticised. Emmelkamp and van der Heyden also point out that most patients in their study "reported an increase of their obsessions during unresolved interpersonal conflict" (1980, p. 33). The obsessions of these patients were therefore considered by these authors to be a result of "*unexpressed* aggressive feelings and the associated guilt" concerning such feelings (1980, p. 29, original emphasis). Emmelkamp and van der Heyden predict that assertion training would help these patients by leading to "a more adequate handling (i.e. expression) of aggression" and by producing a reduction in "guilt feelings and hence [a reduction in] obsessions" (p. 29). Emmelkamp and van der Heyden report that the use of assertion training with these patients led to both an increase in assertive behaviour and a reduction in harming obsessions, and this claim will be examined at some length in Chapter 8.

Janet's suggestion that children who are predisposed to psychasthenia should be encouraged not to avoid confrontations also calls to mind Emmelkamp and van der Heyden's study. Janet's anti-exposure remarks quoted earlier also can be interpreted as consistent with Emmelkamp and van der Heyden's therapeutic approach. Thus, to the extent that harming obsessions may be seen as a symbol of the underlying state of the patient – as being a symbol, that is, of the timidity and unassertiveness of these patients – assertiveness training follows Janet's prescription. Rather than aiming treatment directly at this symbol – as would be done, for example, in exposure therapy – assertiveness training addresses itself instead to the underlying state of these patients (although clearly Emmelkamp and van der Heyden would regard harming obsessions as a product, rather than a symbol, of unassertiveness).

The account of harming obsessions offered by Emmelkamp and van der Heyden is very like the one that Havens (1966) and Pitman (1987a) put forward. Emmelkamp and van der Heyden suggest that feelings of guilt concerning both aggressive feelings and the expression of such feelings ("conflict", in Haven's and Pitman's terms, over such feelings and their expression) produce the patient's unassertive behaviour. Would, then, the successful use of assertion training with these patients – the intervention suggested by Emmelkamp and van der Heyden on the basis of their account of harming obsessions – favour Havens's and Pitman's explanation (see Sections 4.5.4 and 4.5.5) of the genesis of such symptoms over Janet's? It appears not. Janet's account of the harming obsessions of Emmelkamp and van der Heyden's patients would not have been very different from that offered by these authors or by Pitman and Havens. Janet, too, would have suggested that these obsessions are an effect of the timidity of these patients and that acting in a more assertive manner would have reduced the severity of these patients' symptoms. Perhaps Janet would have assigned guilt a less important role in the distress of these patients than the role given it by Emmelkamp and van der Heyden. But even if this is true, this part of Emmelkamp and van der Heyden's account plays no part in formulating their prediction that assertiveness training should help patients with harming obsessions (see Chapter 8).

The situation would evidently be different if assertiveness training were shown to be effective in helping those patients of Janet's who reported feelings of detestation towards their fiances – or if, at least, assertiveness training were shown to be effective in reducing the doubts these patients have concerning their love for their fiances and/or in reducing their inability to feel love for them. Janet's account suggests that in such cases it is because of the patient's inability to feel or express *tender* emotions that she experiences feelings of detestation and that these patients may therefore be contrasted in this respect with those treated by Emmelkamp and van der Heyden – the latter's symptoms were hypothesised by these authors to result from a failure to express anger. Encouraging Janet's patients to express hostile emotion should not, therefore, according to Janet's account, affect their difficulties in experiencing or expressing tender emotions – the patient's hostile emotion is considered a mere effect of these difficulties and its expression would not be predicted, therefore, to be of help in alleviating them.

This prediction distinguishes Janet's account from one that would be defended by Havens (1966) and Pitman (1987a). They suggest that the patient's detestation for her fiance produces her doubts about, and her inability to experience fully, her love for him. If this detestation were in turn hypothesised to be a result of the patient's inability to express hostile emotion appropriately – that is, her not behaving in a sufficiently assertive manner – then it *would* be predicted that an intervention that attempted to promote more assertive behaviour might help alleviate the patient's difficulties in experiencing, or in being sure about, tender feelings.

Janet's account may also be distinguished from one that claims that the primary difficulty of patients such as those treated by Emmelkamp and van der Heyden is that these patients are abnormally angry, their timidity and unassertive manner being explained as their reaction to (or their compensation for) this abnormal degree of anger. Such an account, in contrast to Janet's, would be contradicted by the successful use of assertion training. Suppose there were evidence that adopting ordinary levels of assertiveness is therapeutic for patients with harming obsessions (see Chapter 8). An account of these symptoms in terms of the patients' having an abnormal level of anger appears to predict that similarly abnormal levels of assertiveness or aggression would be necessary for a significant reduction in the severity and frequency of obsessions.

4.8   Summary of comments of Janet

Pitman praises the "clinical astuteness" of Janet's work (Pitman, 1987a, p. 231) and suggests that it is not so much Janet's *theory* of psychasthenia but rather his observations and treatment suggestions concerning the disorder that have stood the test of time. Janet's theory of psychological tension and his speculations as to a physiological tension corresponding to it are, according to Pitman, an unsuccessful attempt to make sense of Janet's observations concerning psychasthenic patients. Some of these observations, however, such as those concerning the interpersonal difficulties encountered by these patients and the co-morbidity of the various symptoms they report, remain important contributions. In the light of Reed's interpretation, it needs to be added that opinions differ on how Janet's theory of psychasthenia is to be understood, but this is not a reason to question Pitman's lack of confidence in the theory. Reed's own account of OCD, which, as noted earlier, has much in common with his interpretation of Janet, meets with substantial difficulties (see Chapter 6). It is of interest that some of Pitman's suggestions as to the nature of OCD, made while outlining a cybernetic model of the disorder, have some similarities with Reed's account. It has also been noted that the account of some symptom contents, to which Janet was led by his theory of psychological tension, may have been too readily rejected by Pitman and Havens. An account similar to Pitman's and Haven's psychodynamic positions on the one hand, and an account similar to Janet's on the other, might provide contrasting predictions about the likely outcome of using assertion training with some (but not all) of the psychasthenic patients described by Janet.

Doubts have been raised about whether Janet's treatment suggestions can be interpreted as a recommendation to use exposure with response prevention with OCD patients. Concerning Janet's clinical observations, doubts have also been raised as to the extent to which these apply to all OCD patients. Nonetheless, some of the observations that Janet provides may well be of importance in making sense of, and even in providing treatments for, some cases of OCD.

4.9   Pitman's cybernetic model of OCD

4.9.1   The principle of a control system

Pitman subjects "aspects of obsessive-compulsive disorder...and related psychopathology to a cybernetic, or control systems, analysis", doing so in the light of Janet's (1903) observation that OCD patients experience their mental activity as incomplete (Pitman,1987a; unless otherwise stated, all Section 4.9 references are to this article; also see Section 4.2). Pitman suggests (p. 334) that his analysis of OCD in terms of cybernetics, a component of modern neuroscience unavailable to Janet, will complement Janet's account of the disorder. As noted in Section 4.5.4, Reed (1985, pp. 176–7) also discusses the relevance of cybernetic theory to Janet's account of OCD.

Central to the cybernetic approach to behaviour, Pitman points out, is its claim that the "organism constitutes a complex control system which attempts to control not its behavioural output...but rather its input or perception, through a negative feedback process" (p. 334). He illustrates the principle of a control system with the example of a thermostat. An internal comparator mechanism detects a mismatch between a perceptual signal (the ambient temperature reading) and a reference signal (the thermostat's setting) and generates an error signal. This causes the activation of behavioural output (the turning on of the heating system) in order to shift the perceptual signal in the direction of the reference signal. This continues until the mismatch between the perceptual and reference signals is eliminated, at which point the error signal becomes zero and the behavioural output stops.

The behaviour of a human being may be similarly understood, Pitman suggests. He gives as an example a person adjusting a thermostat. This behaviour may be seen, Pitman suggests, as resulting from the person's comparator calculating the difference between "an internal comfort perceptual signal and an internal comfort reference signal". This leads to the generation of "an internal error signal, which represents [the person's] discomfort" (p. 335). This causes the person to adjust the thermostat until his discomfort (internal error signal) is eliminated. Pitman notes that different control systems within the same individual may conflict. This is so when a person wants two incompatible goals; in such circumstances, it will be impossible for that person's error signals regarding both of these goals to be simultaneously at zero.

4.9.2 *Pitman's general remarks regarding the cybernetic model*

Pitman's cybernetic model of OCD actually consists of what he presents as three different suggestions regarding the nature of this disorder. Before introducing these suggestions, Pitman offers some remarks concerning the cybernetic approach to behaviour. Pitman suggests that psychological theories in general, and behavioural theories rooted in traditional stimulus–response (S–R) psychology in particular, have had only limited success in explaining OCD because, "uninformed by cybernetics...[they do not take into consideration] the systematic interaction of perception, purpose and overt action" (p. 335) that characterises all behaviour, including that observed in OCD. Pitman considers that the control systems theory, by contrast, "offers unique explanatory possibilities for OCD" (p. 336). He hypothesises that "the core problem in OCD is the persistence of high error signals, or mismatch, that cannot be reduced to zero through behavioural output" (p. 336), and he presents a number of examples of OCD symptoms, including perfectionism and indecision, that, he argues, can be understood in this way.

Pitman proposes that this model could be tested experimentally by tasks requiring OCD patients and controls to report the degree of mismatch they perceive in different classes (for example, auditory, visual, tactile) of paired stimuli. The model predicts, Pitman suggests, that OCD patients will be more inclined than controls to detect mismatch between pairs of stimuli.

Pitman adds to his analysis some speculations as to how it might be applied to current neuroanatomical hypotheses of OCD. He notes that Gray (1982) suggests a role for the septo-hippocampal system and associated limbic areas in OCD, postulating that these areas function to compare predicted to actual events, taking control of behavioural output when mismatch is detected. Pitman finds this analysis similar to his own, although he notes that the emphasis in Gray's work is upon *predictions* or *expectations* rather than, as in Pitman's analysis, *intentions* as reference signals for behaviour (see Section 3.6.1).

Before considering Pitman's three accounts of OCD, one should first note that many of the claims of the cybernetic approach, as presented by Pitman, appear to be entirely uncontroversial. For example, this approach, as Pitman emphasises, conceives of behaviour as *purposeful,* as being performed in order to bring about certain desired states of affairs, rather than (as in S–R psychology) "as simply...learned or innate responses to instigating stimuli" (p. 335). This is, indeed, what Pitman's suggestion that "perception, purpose and overt action interact in all behaviour" really amounts to. But this claim is not one that would be denied as regards the compulsive behaviour of OCD patients, even by behavioural theorists of the disorder such as, for example, Rachman and Hodgson (1980). Similarly, the suggestion that error signals or the perception of mismatch produces compulsive behaviour is not in itself substantive, only amounting to the claim that this behaviour is produced by thoughts such as "X is not perfectly clean" and by any discomfort that the patient experiences in association with such thoughts.

4.9.3   The three accounts presented by Pitman

4.9.3.1   The faulty internal comparator account

Pitman suggests that in the case of some OCD patients, difficulty results from a "faulty internal comparator" – no matter what "perceptual input [the patient's comparator] receives", Pitman suggests, "it continues to register mismatch ...[and thus] while the obsessive-compulsive often feels that an action wasn't done well or completely, to an observer it may appear perfectly well done" (p. 340).

These remarks are open to different interpretations. There are at least two quite different faults that an OCD patient's internal comparator could be hypothesised to have developed:

Hypothesis (1): The error signals generated by the comparator are exceptionally difficult to extinguish.

Hypothesis (2): The error signals are exceptionally strong.

(It is unclear which of these interpretations Pitman would accept.) These two hypotheses need to be carefully distinguished. Hypothesis (1) differs from most other accounts of OCD – including hypothesis (2) – by the fact that it regards as *primary* the difficulty the patient has in dismissing, for example, thoughts that checking or cleaning tasks have not been properly done. Hypothesis (1) suggests that it is this difficulty that *causes* the distress observed, this approach holding in particular that the distress is not produced because thoughts of not having properly cleaned or of having made a mistake are more aversive for the OCD patient than they are for others. Thus, hypothesis (1) would, for example, deny that it *matters* more to the OCD patient whether or not he has been contaminated or made a mistake – it is rather that he only finds it more difficult to establish whether cleaning or checking tasks have been properly performed. This is what is meant here by the faulty comparator's producing signals that are difficult to extinguish, as opposed to signals that are exceptionally strong.

This hypothesis has some similarities to that put forward by Reed (1985, 1990; also see Chapter 6), although Pitman makes, in contrast to Reed, some attempt to explain obsessional impulses (see Pitman, p. 338; also see Section 6.6.1). According to Reed, obsessional disorders are primarily cognitive in nature, the thinking style of the patient, by this approach, hypothesised to produce the patient's discomfort.

A number of difficulties that can be raised for Reed's account (see Chapter 6) may also be brought against hypothesis (1). Two of the most important of these difficulties will be mentioned here. Firstly, there have been numerous studies that have used tasks very like those suggested by Pitman, in which the degree of mismatch perceived by OCD patients has been tested; these studies have failed to substantiate hypothesis (1). (See Section 6.8; although also see Section 4.9.3.3 for a reply Pitman might make to this point.)

Secondly, as was stressed earlier, hypothesis (1) implies, along with Reed's account, that the outcomes of cleaning or checking tasks, for example, should not matter more to the OCD patient than they do to others; the OCD patient differs from other people, according to hypothesis (1), only in being less able to establish that satisfactory outcomes to such tasks have been achieved. Yet this implication is implausible. Many normals, for example, are able to tolerate the possibility, and even indeed the certainty, that their hands have not been properly cleaned or that doors and switches have not been properly checked. It cannot, therefore, merely be the hypothesised difficulty of the OCD patient in establishing that such tasks have been properly done that is the cause of his difficulties on these tasks.

The distress and compulsive behaviour exhibited by an OCD patient can only be explained by a *greater intolerance* of the thoughts that his hands might not have been, or are not, properly washed and that doors and switches might not have been or have not been properly checked, and no account of this greater intolerance is provided by hypothesis (1). This account fails to explain the *motivation* of OCD patients (see Section 6.3 for a fuller statement of this objection).

This difficulty in explaining the motivation of OCD patients is not encountered by hypothesis (2), if the exceptionally strong error signals postulated by this hypothesis are understood to correspond to the OCD patient's experiencing more anxiety (or some other discomfort) at the thought that, for example, his hands have not been properly washed, or doors and switches have not been properly checked. But an account of OCD must surely tell us *why*, not merely *that*, this is so. And there appears to be nothing in Pitman's faulty internal comparator discussion that attempts to meet this requirement.

A further point is worth noting. As mentioned earlier, Pitman suggests that his account to some extent overlaps with Gray's, and this claim is most likely made with the "faulty internal comparator" section of Pitman's discussion in mind. But the interpretation of that section of his discussion referred to as hypothesis (1) is readily distinguishable from Gray's account due to its implying that the outcomes of cleaning and checking tasks, for example, should not matter more to OCD patients than to others. Though encountering difficulties of its own (see Section 3.6), Gray's account clearly states that OCD patients should experience more anxiety than others regarding the tasks that trouble them, and therefore his account has no problem explaining why these tasks matter more to OCD patients. Therefore, if hypothesis (1) is a correct interpretation of Pitman's remarks, his account evidently has less in common with Gray's than Pitman believes.

4.9.3.2 The attentional disturbance account

Pitman suggests that in some OCD patients there may be an "attentional disturbance" involving a "diminished capacity to withdraw attention from...discrepant perceptual signals" (p. 340). It is unclear how this difficulty, thus stated, could be distinguished from the patient's having a faulty internal comparator, the error signals from which are either difficult to extinguish or exceptionally strong. Perhaps the claim would be that the patient's attentional disturbance will also be evident elsewhere in his functioning. But Pitman does not attempt to fill out his suggestion in this or any other way, and so for the purposes of the present discussion, the attentional disturbance and faulty internal comparator hypotheses will be treated as indistinguishable.

4.9.3.3 The conflict/displacement account

Pitman is explicit that he does not intend the faulty internal comparator or attentional disturbance accounts to be the usual ways in which his cybernetic approach is applied. The application he most favours is within a conflict/displacement account, this being the account, Pitman believes, that provides the most plausible explanation of most cases of OCD. Pitman argues that cybernetics can help illuminate such an account because it suggests that conflict results from two control systems' having different reference signals for the same input or perception. One example Pitman gives is a patient's wanting both to confront and not to confront his boss. The problem is thus a matter of "intrapsychic conflict" (p. 339), with compulsive rituals hypothesised to represent the displacement activity that results from this conflict (also see Sections 4.5.4 and 4.5.5).

But how significant a contribution can cybernetic theory make within such an account as this? Neither the notion of intrapsychic conflict nor that of displacement is supposed by Pitman to have been introduced by cybernetics. According to Pitman, the notion of displacement is found in the work of Janet (to whom cybernetics was unavailable) and both the notion of displacement and that of intrapsychic conflict are found in the work of Freud, to whom cybernetics was similarly unavailable (p. 228). All that remains for the cybernetic approach to contribute within this account, therefore, is the observation that the competing behaviours involved in the putative conflict are purposeful. But this appears to be an entirely uncontroversial claim. All theorists would accept that *if* conflict of the type Pitman is discussing here is involved in producing OCD, then such conflict will be between purposes the patient has. Cybernetics, it can be concluded, cannot make any important contribution to the conflict/displacement account of OCD.

What, then, of the conflict/displacement account itself and, in particular, of the suggestion that intrapsychic conflict causes some cases of OCD (also see Section 4.5.5)? This suggestion is not supported by the cases that Pitman (1987a) cites as illustrating the role that conflict plays in OCD. He presents, for example, the case of a patient who experienced difficulty in choosing between two desired options on a menu. Unable to decide which of the options he wanted most, the patient would vacillate between them for prolonged periods of time. But this does not show that conflict was involved in *causing* such a symptom in the manner required by Pitman's conflict/displacement account or that this patient's indecisiveness is a *displacement* of any putative conflict. The conflict to which reference is being made here is *part of* the symptom; thus, to say that the patient's difficulties with menus involves conflict of this kind is just a description of the problem, rather than a causal claim. Similarly, nothing here suggests that any behaviour that cannot be attributed to either of two competing inclinations (see Section 4.5.4) has been produced by the conflict involved – which is the suggested role for conflict in Pitman's conflict/displacement account. And it seems, therefore, that once again Pitman's cybernetic approach cannot tell us anything further about problems such as this patient's difficulties with menus other than the fact that such a problem involves the patient's harbouring competing desires or intentions. And yet this much is, once again, surely already evident merely from a description of the patient's difficulties.

As regards those cases in which Pitman hypothesises the conflict/displacement account to apply, he is explicit that one need not postulate structural abnormality with either control system (that is, with either of those hypothesised to be in conflict). His position is thus explicitly that there is only an intrinsic comparator defect in *some* cases of OCD, which appears to require some qualification of his prediction (p. 339) that it should be possible to show that OCD patients differ from controls when asked to report their perceived degree of mismatch concerning paired stimuli in laboratory tasks. Indeed, Pitman introduces his hypothesis of an intrinsic comparator defect only after stating that "it is tempting to hypothesise that all [obsessive-compulsive] psychopathology is caused by underlying conflict", but then conceding that "a causative role for conflict is difficult to establish in all cases" (p. 340). According to these remarks, Pitman's prediction as regards the performance of OCD patients on the laboratory tasks he proposes would apply only to a minority of such patients and would thus enable him to explain laboratory findings such as those discussed in Section 6.8 (and which were also referred to in Section 4.9.3.1).

Another problem for the conflict/displacement account is that it might not predict that difficulties in matching perceptual and reference signals (that is, difficulties in establishing, for example, that cleaning or checking tasks have been properly done) are evident in compulsive behaviour at all. According to this account, difficulties in matching perceptual and reference signals arise as a result of conflict encountered elsewhere producing compulsive behaviour as a displacement activity. Would the account not predict, therefore, that if severe difficulties in matching perceptual and reference signals are also encountered in the area in which the displacement activity arises, a *second* displacement should occur in response to *these* difficulties, and so on until an activity not involving such difficulties is found? That is, if the *point* of some activity is supposed to be the attempted relief or resolution of difficulties in matching perceptual and reference signals encountered elsewhere in the patient's functioning, it seems that one would not expect this activity itself to involve such matching difficulties. If this is correct, then all of the examples Pitman gives of compulsive behaviour involving difficulties in matching perceptual and reference signals may actually contradict the conflict/displacement account. This, incidentally, suggests an interesting contrast between accounts of compulsive behaviour in terms of *displacement* mechanisms on the one hand, and in terms of *symbolic* mechanisms on the other. Some, if not all, versions of the latter type of account *would* predict that compulsive behaviour reflects the conflict experienced by the patient. (Symbolisation is discussed further in Section 5.4.3.)

4.9.4 Summary of Pitman's cybernetic model

In presenting a cybernetic model of OCD, Pitman discusses a number of interesting cases where symptoms involve indecisiveness, perfectionism and conflict. But, insofar as the cybernetic model makes substantive suggestions concerning the explanation of OCD – in terms of a fault in the postulated internal comparator mechanism that makes error signals more difficult to extinguish – it encounters a number of difficulties, the most important of these being in making sense of the motivation of patients suffering from the disorder. Insofar as these difficulties are avoided – by supposing the internal comparator fault to produce error signals that are abnormally strong, or by presenting the cybernetic model within a conflict/displacement account – it appears that the cybernetic component of these accounts fails to make any substantive contribution to them. Therefore, it must be concluded that, in its present form, the model does not significantly advance our understanding of OCD.

5   Psychodynamic approaches to OCD

5.1   Introduction

Much of the theorising found in psychodynamic approaches tends to pay close attention to the detail of individual patients. This makes it difficult to review thoroughly the whole of the psychodynamic literature on OCD, and in what follows no attempt to do this will be made. To the extent that generalisations across individual patients are possible from this perspective, furthermore, one finds psychodynamic theorists offering a number of different accounts of OCD. It seems unlikely that each of these is intended to apply to a different subgroup of OCD patients, and these accounts thus stand instead as alternative, and perhaps also incompatible, approaches to the disorder.

Given these points, the present discussion will take the following course. Firstly, some of the psychodynamic accounts of OCD that have been offered will be briefly outlined, the emphasis being on exposition rather than criticism. Following this, a single case discussion presented by Malan (1979) will be critically discussed at some length, along with some of Malan's comments concerning psychodynamic theory and therapy. There are two justifications for concentrating critical comment on Malan's case discussion. Firstly, and as already noted, much psychodynamic theorising takes into account the detail of individual patients and is therefore also best discussed with reference to such details. This does not, of course, mean that all of the points raised by any given case will be irrelevant to the evaluation of psychodynamic accounts of other cases, and indeed, it is suggested that some of the themes raised by the case discussion to be considered here (for example, the nature of symbolisation and the role of the unconscious) would be central to many psychodynamic discussions.

Secondly, Malan's work represents a higher hurdle than most for critics of psychodynamic approaches. For example, he himself offers cogent criticisms of a number of the least plausible aspects of psychodynamic theory, and his work also has the virtue of making clear the precise grounds on which interpretations are being offered. This makes it possible to evaluate these interpretations and to consider alternative explanations of the same clinical data. This clearly contrasts most favourably with those psychodynamic authors who tend instead to offer "intuitive assertions...[which savour] of apostolic vision" (Reed, 1985, p. 186). For example, Reed correctly points out that some of Fenichel's (1977) account is of this variety. Malan's attempts to provide clearly argued formulations of clinical material can be linked to another feature of his work: an interest in the systematic evaluation of the outcome of psychodynamic therapies (Malan, 1976); both of these aspects of

Malan's work can be seen as attempts to exhibit a rational foundation for his psychodynamic work and, as such, are relevant to the still-debated question of whether or not psychodynamic theory may be regarded as a science (Grünbaum, 1986). No attempt to examine this question in any detail will be made, although one or two remarks concerning this are offered at the end of the chapter; some further comments on this and related issues are presented in Chapter 8.

5.2   Some psychodynamic theories of OCD

Probably the best-known psychodynamic account of OCD is that in which Freud attempts to explain the disorder with reference to the psychosexual stages postulated in his account of human development. According to this account, a child's sexuality passes through three stages, being mediated first through the mouth, then the anus and finally the genitals – the oral, anal (or "anal-sadistic") and genital stages. According to Freud (1905), later elaborated in Fenichel's (1977) account, fixation at, and regression to, a particular stage of psychosexual development determine the nature of the disorder that appears in later life. In the case of OCD, one of the putative stages of development involved is the anal stage, although the later phallic stage is also supposed to have a central role.

The supposed "association of traits of cruelty and of anal eroticism in compulsion neurosis" (Fenichel, 1977, p. 273) convinced Freud (1913a) of the existence of an anal-sadistic stage of development. Toilet training is supposed to be of central importance to this developmental stage, with anger, aggression, and the exercise of control over others being associated with it. Fixation at, and regression to, this stage of development are also argued by Freud (1908) to determine the development of the obsessional personality and personality disorders.

What are termed "anal" and "sadistic" impulses are thus supposed to be evident in OCD. Their presence is meant to explain the conflict observed in sufferers over such matters as "aggression and submissiveness, cruelty and gentleness, dirtiness and cleanliness, order and disorder" (Fenichel, 1977, p. 273). The first items in each of these pairs (that is, aggressiveness, cruelty, etc.) are hypothesised to be "direct anal or sadistic outbreaks" (Fenichel, 1977, p. 274); the second items (that is, submissiveness, gentleness, etc.), reaction formations that defend the patient against the tendency to such outbreaks. "Instinctive" and "anti-instinctive" forces (Fenichel, 1977, p. 269) are thus supposed to be at work in OCD, and mixtures of these, this psychodynamic approach suggests, are sometimes observed, producing apparently contradictory patterns of behaviour (for example, the patient's persecuting others with his extreme solicitude or pity).

An apparent contradiction in OCD for this approach is that although it stresses the supposed anal-sadistic phase of development in its account of the disorder, difficulties that putatively stem from the Oedipus complex are commonly observed in OCD patients, according to this same approach (for example, Freud, 1909, 1913a). These difficulties along with other features of OCD – for example, see Fenichel, 1977, p. 274) are associated by this approach with the putative phallic stage, a supposedly later development than the anal-sadistic stage. The attempt to resolve this apparent contradiction stresses the hypothesised role of regression in the disorder. According to Freud, regression to the anal-sadistic stage occurs in these patients in response to the Oedipal crisis, supposedly leading to a mixed profile of Oedipal and anal-sadistic phenomena.

Although the purpose of this brief review section of the present chapter is merely to outline various psychodynamic approaches to OCD, one or two comments on the foregoing account are offered here. Although some of the observations made in setting out this account certainly do seem to apply to some OCD patients – for example, the conflict in some patients over aggressiveness and submissiveness, order and disorder – the absence of evidence supporting Freud's account of psychosexual developmental stages has been frequently noted, for example, by Rachman and Hodgson (1980, pp. 144–5) and Emmelkamp (1982, pp. 182–8, especially pp. 184–6). Malan also accepts that such theorising lacks evidential support, and he rejects, at least in much of his discussion (for example, 1979, p. 185), the importance placed on the parts of the body by Freud's developmental account. Despite this, some of the claims Malan makes regarding the case to be discussed here will require us to return to these suggestions about the role of toilet training – and the hostile emotion that is supposedly associated with it – in the genesis of OCD.

As emphasised at the onset of this chapter, there is no single psychodynamic approach to OCD, and no reference to the supposed anal-sadistic and phallic stages of development is required in presenting other accounts from this perspective. For example, the presence of magical and superstitious thinking in some OCD patients led Freud to compare the mental lives of these patients with those of "savages" (Freud, 1913b) and religious believers (Freud, 1907). These same features have also led to a comparison between OCD patients and children (Ferenczi, 1980) and the suggestion that OCD results from a return to childhood patterns of thinking. It is also pointed out that "promises [of] protection on condition of submission" exist both within "patriarchal religions" (Fenichel, 1977, p. 302) and OCD (where it may be only the patient's own conscience, rather than the will of a god, to which submission is required for the patient to be granted "good luck"); it is further pointed out that there are once again similarities with children, "protection on condition of submission" being given to them by adults, and in particular by their parents. These ideas play no part in the case discussion presented later, and so will not be subject to detailed comment here; nonetheless, the parallels this account points out between some OCD patients and these phenomena of childhood and religious life are undeniably intriguing.

Another psychodynamic approach is offered by Adler (1964), who suggests that OCD and other psychiatric difficulties result from the patient's failing to feel in control of important aspects of his or her life. Adler argues that compulsive behaviour results from an unconscious attempt to compensate for this by achieving mastery over the tasks and situations that feature in that behaviour. There are, as will be seen, certain similarities between this view and the position taken by Malan in the case discussion considered later; he too suggests that control over symptom contents may be sought as a response to failure to achieve a sense of mastery elsewhere. Interestingly, a somewhat similar account is also advanced as part of Rachman and Hodgson's (1980) behavioural account, which suggests that compulsive behaviour may sometimes be a "compensatory rebound" from experiences of helplessness in important situations in the patient's life (p. 394).

Finally, Malan himself, in commenting on the case discussion to be presented here (which he terms the case of the "pesticide chemist"), makes clear that he does not intend this case to be seen as typical of *all* instances of OCD. Malan hypothesises that the problem in this case results from unexpressed anger, but he makes it clear that he should "not wish to give the impression that obsessional symptoms are always a defence against aggressive feelings....[they] can be a defence against any kind of disturbing conflict" (Malan, 1979, p. 109). Malan is certainly correct that one sees cases of OCD quite unlike that of the pesticide chemist. It is worth noting in passing here, for example, that in his account of so-called "primitive phenomena" (Malan, 1979, Chapter 15), Malan discusses the theme of "attacking the good" with respect to a patient (not suffering from OCD) whom he describes as endeavouring to destroy "everything good *of his own*" (Malan, 1979, p. 170, original emphasis). This certainly seems to share something with a phenomenon one observes in some cases of OCD – a tendency for symptoms to arise in, and to wreck, situations and activities that would otherwise be a source of great pleasure for the patient. Such features as these seem less readily observed in the case of the pesticide chemist.

Before discussing this case, some background detail and comment regarding Malan's general views on psychodynamic theory and therapy will be offered.

5.3   Malan on psychodynamic theory and therapy

5.3.1   *Psychodynamic explanations and the "act of insight"*

According to Malan, a psychodynamic therapist should (1) indicate how the factors that precipitate a given symptom suggest the putative conflict that is supposed to be expressed or represented by that symptom and (2) provide a detailed mechanism whereby this expression or representation has occurred. Interpreting this mechanism to the patient, Malan further suggests, should (3) "bring the conflict clearly into consciousness" and this in turn should (4) "result in the disappearance of the symptom" (Malan, 1979, p. 107). Malan thus argues that therapeutic change in psychodynamic therapy *directly results from* the bringing of conflict into consciousness.

Malan also acknowledges (1979, pp. 218–19) that psychodynamic therapies have had little success with OCD and argues, contrary to his general account of psychodynamic therapy, that when "obsessional symptoms, and particularly obsessional rituals" are treated by psychotherapy, "everything becomes intelligible and the patient becomes conscious of the conflict, but therapeutic results do not ensue" (Malan, 1979, p. 107). Malan argues that a major challenge for psychodynamic theories of OCD is the explanation of the positive effects of behaviour therapy with this disorder (p. 107; also see Section 8.2).

Not all psychodynamic theorists would accept Malan's account of psychodynamic therapy, particularly his suggestion that therapeutic effects are the direct result of bringing conflicts into consciousness. Symington, for example, would regard such an account as giving "too much weight to the act of insight" (Symington, 1985, p. 26) and would suggest that this picture is contrary to the whole psychodynamic conception of people as "ruled by the irrational". He instead suggests insight to be an effect of change in psychotherapy and argues that "emotional change and insight are manifestations of things going on at a deeper level of the psyche" (p. 26).

Malan also suggests that conditions (1)–(4) are in certain respects similar to "Koch's postulates" by which one can judge whether a given disease is caused by a particular bacterium (Malan, 1979, p. 107).

5.3.2 *Evidence relevant to psychodynamic formulations*

Malan presents "four categories of evidence" as providing potential support for any psychodynamic formulation (1979, p. 55). The first three of his categories restate the four conditions Malan discusses as being in certain respects similar to "Koch's postulates", and Malan adds to them another possible line of evidence, which he describes as "the patient's response to interpretations". By this he means whether or not the interpretation deepens the rapport between the patient and therapist. There is an asymmetry in Malan's discussion of this point. He suggests that an interpretation may be "inappropriate" – that is, reduce rapport – while being perfectly true. This will be so, for example, if the patient is not ready to accept the interpretation, Malan suggests. But this raises the question of whether or not *false* interpretations may sometimes deepen rapport because, for example, they happen to be merely what the patient wants to hear. Malan does not discuss this point but does frequently use, in his case discussions, an interpretation's deepening rapport as confirmatory evidence for the validity of that interpretation. He evidently holds, therefore, that it is very unlikely that false interpretations could have this effect (see Section 5.5.5[b]).

5.3.3 *The two triangles*

Malan divides interpretations into two categories, those concerning what he calls the *triangle of conflict* and those concerning what he calls the *triangle of person*. Malan suggests that almost every interpretation can be presented in terms of one or both of these two triangles.

Malan describes the triangle of conflict as consisting of the patient's defence, anxiety and hidden feeling. Examples of each of these will be provided later in the case discussion. The triangle of person consists of what

Malan calls "other", "transference" and "parent". (*Other* is usually used to refer to relationships with people in the patient's current life or recent past – such as a marriage partner or close friend; *transference* refers to the relationship between the patient and therapist.) It is in his relationships with people in all three of these categories that the patient's triangle of conflict is supposed to occur. The same defence, anxiety and hidden feeling, that is, should be at work in all of these relationships, Malan suggests, and the aim of psychotherapy, according to Malan, is to help the patient trace them back from the present (the "other" and "transference" relationships) to the past (the relationship with the parent[s]). The feelings that were directed toward the parent(s) are supposed by Malan to be *the reason for* the feelings that are found in the present relationships. The feelings in these present relationships are thus seen as co-effects of this common cause.

Elsewhere, Malan (1976) presents statistical evidence that suggests that those therapies in which what are supposed to be the patient's hidden feelings regarding his or her parents are reached are the therapies that also tend to be the most successful. Further evidence would, of course, be required to show that it is *because* of this that these therapies are successful.

5.4   The case of the pesticide chemists

5.4.1   *Malan's account of the pesticide chemist*

The pesticide chemist is described by Malan (1979, pp. 101–7) as an overconscientious person suffering from what Malan describes as three obsessional symptoms:

> "(i) perfectionism, which he finds it difficult to maintain e.g. in relation to the assistants working under him;
> (ii) need to keep things tidy, which he also cannot maintain; and
> (iii) obsessional anxiety, in the form of a preoccupation with the fear that he may not have done his work properly" (Malan 1979, p. 102).

Despite his efforts at work, the patient is reported not to have received much appreciation from his boss and also to have clashed with his wife over the amount of time he spends at work. He is further described as always having suffered from premature ejaculation and as having been mildly depressed for the few months prior to referral.

Things came to a head, Malan reports, when the patient's wife suggested one morning that he spend a day at home due to his low mood. He chose instead to set off for work, so his wife said that she would in that case get on with treating the house for woodworm. This was a job that he had been working on himself for a year or so, and he subsequently reported to his therapist that he took this remark of his wife's as an implicit criticism of his efforts in this regard. His response was an uncharacteristic outburst of rage, during which he tipped the antiwoodworm solution down the sink, struck his wife, and finally cried for some hours.

It is worth noting here that this patient, contrary to Malan's account, might not be suffering from obsessional *symptoms* at all. He is reported to have sought help regarding only his loss of energy, his depression and his outburst of rage. It might be argued, then, that what are described as his symptoms may only be the operation of obsessional *traits*; however, following Malan's intervention, features (i)–(iii) are reported, as will be seen, to have entirely disappeared, indicating that Malan may be correct on this point after all.

5.4.2 The triangle of conflict for the pesticide chemist

Malan points out that, with respect to both his boss and his wife, the patient reported that he encountered his best efforts' being met with criticism. Malan also notes that running through the patient's three symptoms is the theme of *precariously keeping something at bay* (1979, p. 102, original emphasis) – namely the patient's own and others' potential mistakes. Malan brings these pieces of evidence together and adds to them a third – that when the patient does have a breakdown, this takes the form of an intense outburst of rage.

In the light of these points, Malan raises the question of whether "all three of these obsessional symptoms are symbolic ways of *controlling angry feelings*" (p. 102, original emphasis). This, then, gives us the triangle of conflict for this patient: "the *defence* is symbolic control, while the *anxiety* is his fear of the harm he may do if he expresses the *hidden feeling*, which is anger" (Malan, 1979, pp. 102–3, original emphasis).

The suggestion that the demands that others are placing upon this patient may be of importance to understanding his problems seems to be given some support by the subsequent developments in his therapy. His hypothesised anger at these demands, Malan tells us, is "brought into consciousness", with the result that the patient is able to resist the demands that are being made upon him and become angry with people when necessary. His obsessional symptoms are reported to have disappeared at two-month follow-up, this situation being maintained at a further follow-up nearly four years later, in contrast to what Malan describes as the usual outcome of psychodynamic treatment with OCD patients. Malan does not provide here, however, experimentally controlled findings in favour of the hypothesis that encouraging this patient to resist the demands of others was a crucial ingredient in his therapy. Indeed, there is at present very little evidence that encouraging OCD patients to do this is helpful (see Section 4.7.3 and Chapter 8).

5.4.3 The triangle of person for the pesticide chemist

Turning to the triangle of person, Malan asks where the anger, which he suggests to be apparent in this patient's various current relationships, has originated and suggests that it goes back to this patient's parents, and in particular his father. It seems that the father was constantly away from home earning money for the family, rendering him someone "with whom it was impossible to be angry" (Malan, 1979, p. 103) despite the father's lengthy and sorely felt absences. It is this,

Malan suggests, "which is likely to have set up a conflict in him [the patient] about whether he should express his anger and make demands on his own behalf, or control his anger and meet the demands of his environment" (p. 103).

5.5   Evaluation of the psychodynamic aspects of this case discussion

5.5.1   Introduction

In virtue of which features might Malan's account of the pesticide chemist's difficulties be said to be psychodynamic in nature? There are at least four features that might be argued to give it this character – its referring to unconscious mental processes; its referring to symbolic mechanisms; its explanation of the reported symptoms as having arisen in order to serve the patient's purposes; and its suggestion that the patient's achieving insight, and particularly insight into his childhood relationship with his parents, is central to the treatment of the patient's difficulties. Each of these features will now be considered in turn.

5.5.2   The "unconscious"

There are many references in Malan's account to unconscious emotions' being at work – specifically anger and the anxiety that is hypothesised to be provoked by it – and it might be thought that this helps to characterise his account as psychodynamic. There is, however, no need to reify "the unconscious" in order to make sense of these references. One need only assert that the patient is not in perfect touch with his own emotions or, put in other words, is not fully aware of these emotions. Malan claims both (1) that the patient is angry but not aware of his own anger and (2) that the patient is anxious, but wrongly believes this anxiety to have been caused by tasks at home and at work, when in reality he is anxious about being angry. Couching these two claims in terms of the patient's not being in touch with, or not being fully aware of, his own emotions is not merely to state his putative problems in a different way. The claim that people may not be in touch with their own feelings and the claim that this may sometimes lead them into difficulties surely seem, once couched in these terms, to be pieces of common sense (also see Ryle, 1949, Chapter 4). If there is, then, anything distinctively psychodynamic about Malan's reference to unconscious processes, this is at most merely a semantic matter. This is not in itself, of course, confirmation of Malan's formulation of the pesticide chemist's problems. But if this formulation is to be rejected, it cannot be on the grounds that the unconscious does not exist. The use of such phrases as the patient's "not being fully aware of" his own emotions also leads one very readily to think that there are degrees to which this may be the case. A dichotomous distinction between conscious and unconscious processes might perhaps be thought to imply, in contrast, that this distinction is not a question of degree (an implication that would probably be unwelcome to writers such as Malan).

5.5.3 Symbolisation

Malan makes use of the notions of symbol, symbolic control, and so forth in his discussion of the case of the pesticide chemist. He argues that the feature of "being precariously kept at bay" is shared by both the patient's anger, on the one hand, and the task demands he perceives himself to face at home and work, on the other. It is this shared feature that Malan cites in claiming that these perceived task demands *symbolise* the patient's anger for him, rendering his attempts to meet these perceived task demands symbolic ways of controlling his angry feelings. This shared feature can surely not, however, be in itself sufficient to justify the claim that perceived task demands symbolise the patient's anger, and it is perhaps not entirely clear on what grounds Malan himself thinks this claim is justified. Other than there being a shared feature, in terms of which one thing may be said to symbolise another, what else is implied by speaking of symbolisation, symbolic control, and so on, in the present (that is, psychiatric) context? It might be argued that another implication is that, to take the example of the pesticide chemist, this patient's hypothesised anxiety as regards his own anger has in some sense *become* his anxiety about perceived task demands and his hypothesised anger has in some sense similarly *become* his perception of those task demands. If reference to symbolisation is to be justified, it is not sufficient, according to this argument, that the patient should have merely *mistakenly attributed* his anxiety about one thing (his anger) to something else (perceived task demands) that is in some respect similar to his anger. It must, rather, be the case that his anxiety as regards that which is being symbolised (his anxiety about his anger) has *turned into* anxiety about that by which his anger is symbolised (anxiety about perceived task demands) and, similarly, that that which is being symbolised (anger) has *turned into* that by which it is symbolised (perceptions of task demands).

It is worth noting that the hypothesised process of converting emotion about one thing into emotion about something else, and the hypothesised process of converting emotion into perceptions of task demands, seem as if they might be of some use or help to the patient, whereas the process of merely wrongly attributing emotion probably does not. Thus, in the case of the pesticide chemist, these hypothesised processes of converting emotion would seem to enable the patient to gain some control over his emotions by meeting the task demands he perceives.

Does the foregoing imply that there is some tension between Malan's referring to this patient's anger as being symbolised, on the one hand, and as being unconscious, on the other? Describing the patient's anger as being unconscious was suggested in the foregoing discussion to mean that "the patient is angry, but does not realise that this is so". Yet, after the hypothesised symbolisation has taken place, is it not, on the foregoing account of symbolisation, correct to say that the patient is no longer angry at all? And that he can thus not now be unconsciously angry, on the foregoing account of the unconscious? Yet it seems paradoxical, from a psychodynamic point of view, to say that an emotion cannot be both unconscious and symbolised at the same time. Perhaps, however, the present discussion does not make it necessary to say this. After all, it is still the case, on the present interpretation of Malan's remarks, that the explanation of the patient's becoming concerned about task demands is that he had been angry, and this anger may thus still be said to be what, in some sense, his concern for task demands is "really about".

To say that Malan's use of the term *symbolisation* implies that these processes of converting emotion are taking place is, of course, not to say that there is any good reason for supposing these processes to take place. Why, then, should one suppose that they are taking place in the case of the pesticide chemist? And what is one to make of Malan's claim that there are similarities between the stresses and symptoms observed in this case? At least two independent criticisms of Malan's position seem plausible.

Firstly, consider Malan's claims of similarities between the hypothesised precipitants of the pesticide chemist's symptoms and the symptoms themselves. A problem for Malan here is that there will always be *some* similarity between *any* precipitating stress (or situation) and *any* symptom, a fact to which some philosophers of science – most notably Popper (1963, 1972) – have drawn attention in criticising psychoanalytic work. If symbolic meaning can in this way "explain" *any* symptomatic response to *any* stress, then it is evidently not explaining anything at all.

Related to this first criticism is the observation that unexpressed anger is hypothesised by Malan to be the precipitating problem in very many cases that, in contrast to the case of the pesticide chemist, do not involve difficulties in which the theme of "precariously keeping something at bay" is observed at all (1979, pp. 95–6, Table 2). In some of these cases, Malan is admirably straightforward in saying that nobody knows why a certain stress sometimes gives rise to a given symptom. For example, in the case of the "drama student" (1979, pp. 33–4), Malan hypothesises that unexpressed anger (and jealousy) have given rise to a fear of travelling underground, a link that Malan declares to be mysterious. But is it not plain that this link could be easily explained in symbolic terms? Why not, for example, suppose that this patient's fear of travelling underground is her way of "symbolically avoiding" emotions she has repressed – that is, emotions she has "forced underground", as one might metaphorically express it? It is indeed the very ease, as just illustrated, with which such suggestions can be made that is the problem for this approach.

Secondly, Malan argues for a symbolic connection between various aspects of the pesticide chemist's life and his obsessional difficulties, without paying due attention to alternative explanations. Indeed, an alternative explanation is implicit in some of Malan's own remarks. Thus, the pesticide chemist is angry, Malan argues, because he is trying to please everyone by performing tasks to perfection and by attempting to have them so performed by his subordinates (see Section 5.4.2). Is it not, therefore, far more straightforward to suppose that the pesticide chemist's precarious efforts to keep task demands at bay are the *source*, rather than the *symbol*, of this patient's anger? On this supposition, it is because of perceived unreasonable demands at home and work that the pesticide chemist is both anxious and angry – anxious that he may not be able to meet all of these demands, and angry that they have been placed upon him. Malan's intervention, it might be argued, is helpful because it enables the patient, through his greater assertiveness, to exercise effective control over these perceived task demands at home and work, which are a genuine source of stress for him. It appears, therefore, that there is no necessity to hypothesise any symbolic connection to make sense either of the difficulties of the pesticide chemist, or of his reported progress in therapy.

5.5.4 The patient's purposes

The third feature that might be argued to give Malan's discussion a psychodynamic character is the manner in which it aims to make sense of the pesticide chemist's difficulties in terms of his purposes. Malan sees the patient as *trying* both to avoid and to control his own anger. *In order to achieve these ends*, Malan suggests, the patient is both not acknowledging his anger, and subjecting it to symbolic control. Both the pesticide chemist's lack of awareness concerning his emotional state, and his obsessional difficulties, are thus seen as things that the patient *has done or produced*, not things that have *happened to* him. In the discussion that follows, attention will focus on the claim that the patient has produced his lack of awareness concerning his own emotional state.

Let it be allowed, then, that the pesticide chemist is, as Malan suggests, out of touch with his own anger when he presents for treatment. Malan appears just to assume, given this, that the patient has *produced* this state of affairs – Malan suggests that we must accept this if we do not merely dismiss the patient's problems "as something mysterious for which there is no point in looking for an explanation" and instead "take them seriously and try to explain them in terms of intelligible human anxieties" (1979, p. 102). Yet given the complexity of some emotional reactions, one clearly cannot just *assume* that the patient has produced his lack of awareness of his own anger. Why can it not be simple error that causes a person not to understand the emotions he or she is experiencing? (Klein's account of *splitting* in neonates has been criticised on broadly similar grounds by A. Ryle, personal communication, 1990.)

Why should Malan assume that it *cannot* be simple error? Maybe one influence on this, discussed by Ryle (1949, especially Chapter 4), is the tendency to think that people have a privileged access to their own emotions and motives – much as they might be argued to have such an access, for example, to their own aches and pains. (A closely allied tendency is to think that people also have incorrigible knowledge of their own emotions and motives.) The possession of such access might be thought to imply that whenever somebody's honest self-report demonstrated an ignorance of his or her own emotions or motives, this could only be because of self-deception on the part of that person – that is, because the person has failed to face something that he or she knows to be true.

Against such a position, it need only be remarked that Ryle correctly points out that we have no privileged access (or incorrigible knowledge) of our own emotions and motives, and such access cannot, therefore, provide grounds for what seems to be Malan's implicit assumption that people must always have some reason for not being fully aware of their own emotions and motives.

5.5.5 Insight

The fourth feature that arguably helps to make Malan's work recognisably psycho-dynamic is his treatment recommendations. As discussed earlier, he sees insight as being the motor of change in therapy and believes the best symptomatic improve-ment to occur as a result of the patient's coming to understand the nature of the hid-den feelings he putatively has toward his parents. The belief in the potency of this kind of insight is at least arguably peculiar to psychoanalytic writers, albeit not shared by all of them (for example, see Symington's remarks quoted earlier).

What evidence is there that insight is important in the case of the pesticide chemist? This question will be considered first as regards the triangle of conflict, and then as regards the triangle of person.

(a) THE TRIANGLE OF CONFLICT
According to Malan's account, the pesticide chemist, during his therapy, became

(1) more aware of his anger concerning a number of things in his life,
(2) more able to give appropriate expression to this anger, and
(3) less handicapped by his obsessional difficulties.

Why does Malan, consistent with his earlier remarks (Section 5.3), take (1) to be the fundamental change (Malan, 1979, p. 108) – especially given the fact that, as noted earlier, he states elsewhere in his discussion (p. 107) that OCD patients may gain insight of this kind without any therapeutic effects? Besides, if it is, as Malan himself argues (1979, pp. 96–7), "constructive assertion" that is supposed to be therapeutic for this patient, it is difficult to see why his merely becoming *aware* that he needs to be more constructively assertive should, by itself, be of help. Similarly, why should the patient's merely being made aware of anger that he is supposed to be anxious about feeling make him less anxious about, and thus more able to express, that anger?

Given these points, then, would it not be more plausible for Malan to suggest that (2) is the most important factor producing condition (3)? The most crucial change for this patient, on this supposition, is not his becoming more aware of his anger, but his becoming more successful in dealing with it (his becoming more appropriately assertive), with his awareness of his own anger perhaps increasing only as a result of his becoming more assertive. (This may indeed be what happened to two of Emmelkamp and van der Heyden's [1980] patients, who appeared to achieve insight into their interpersonal problems only after they had begun assertiveness training; see Section 8.5.)

(b) THE TRIANGLE OF PERSON

Malan does not offer any argument in favour of insight into the triangle of person being important to the pesticide chemist. Thus, despite the favourable therapeutic outcome reported, we are told (Malan, 1979 p. 105) that the pesticide chemist himself has made nothing of the suggestion that his childhood relationship with his father was the origin of his difficulties in resisting the demands of others, and Malan reports that the patient says "he was not aware of such feelings (i.e., unexpressed anger) in his childhood". Furthermore, even if the patient had experienced an improvement in his obsessional difficulties in response to this interpretation concerning his childhood relationship with his father, it is surely clear that this cannot in itself be strong support for the truth of this interpretation, contrary to the third of Malan's four categories of evidence (see Section 5.3). Similarly, if this interpretation had deepened the rapport between the pesticide chemist and his therapist, it is clear that this too would not be in itself confirmation of the truth of this interpretation, contrary to the fourth of Malan's four categories. If our concern is with the truth, rather than with the therapeutic value, of the interpretation concerned, the effects of this interpretation on treatment outcome and/or therapeutic rapport are clearly acceptable tests of the interpretation only on the assumption that the interpretation could not affect the patient in these ways if it were false. And why should one accept this assumption? Is it not, indeed, clear that people can be deeply affected by all manner of false beliefs, and in some cases favourably affected, in the sense of being able to be happier about their lives?

Taking the triangles of person and conflict for the pesticide chemist together, therefore, one may in conclusion state that there is probably no good reason for supposing that insight into either of these hypothesised triangles is of central importance for this patient, contrary to Malan's account of how psychodynamic therapies work in general and of how the pesticide chemist's therapy worked in particular.

It can be further pointed out that other arguments Malan uses provide no good evidence in favour of the patient's childhood relationship with his father being at the root of his difficulties. This claim will be examined in the section that follows.

5.6   The role of childhood experience

Some of the issues discussed by Malan as regards the triangle of conflict for the pesticide chemist raise testable questions. As is argued elsewhere (Chapter 8), for example, the hypothesis that a patient's being insufficiently assertive is contributing to his difficulties lends itself readily to empirical investigation. It is relatively easy to attempt to manipulate the patient's level of assertiveness, and the hypothesis that this is an important factor in the production of his distress has clear implications for the effects that this manipulation, if successful, should have.

The situation regarding the issues raised by the triangle of person for the pesticide chemist (Section 5.4.3) is quite different. It is obviously not possible to manipulate the variables involved here – for example, the past behaviour of the patient's father, the patient's childhood reaction to this behaviour, and so forth – in order to see what effect such manipulations would have upon the patient's present difficulties. How, then, does Malan attempt to support his suggestions about the triangle of person for this patient?

What Malan would perhaps regard as the most important justification of his suggestions is that the relationship between the pesticide chemist and his father should strike us as providing a plausible common-sense explanation of the patient's problems in adult life. The appeal is to our common-sense understanding that "the child is father to the man" and that such childhood experiences will therefore make certain problems in adult life more likely to occur.

How powerful is this appeal in the present case? Part of Malan's argument is that the patient's relationship with his father bears certain similarities to his relationships with his wife and boss. Suppose it be granted for the sake of argument (and contrary to the pesticide chemist's own remarks regarding his relationship with his father) that these similarities do obtain – that all these relationships involve the pesticide chemist's not expressing his angry feelings at what he perceives as the unreasonable treatment he receives. Can these similarities not be explained by considering the pesticide chemist's childhood difficulties with his father to be simply *another instance* of exactly the same character disposition that is observed in this patient as an adult and that produced his difficulties at home and work – that is, his being poor at expressing his feelings and demanding what he wants? Why suppose this disposition to have *originated* in his relationship with his father instead of merely having been *instantiated* there, its cause being more a matter of, for example, innate factors? Malan readily suggests that the patient's behaviour is at the heart of his adult problems, yet Malan appears to overlook entirely the contribution this factor may have made to childhood experiences. If the patient as an adult is said to have relationships in which his feelings are not expressed largely or entirely because of his own behaviour, why should the influence of the patient's behavior be largely or entirely denied as regards the nature of relationships the patient had as a child?

Perhaps in reply to this, and in support of the primary importance of childhood relationships, it might be argued that adults *choose* as their spouses and friends people who resemble their parents. It is, according to this reply, being able to make such choices that (1) is a major reason why adults are able to exercise more control than children over the nature of the important relationships in their lives and (2) is how – in influencing or determining these adult choices –

childhood relationships are of primary importance. Perhaps, then, as regards the pesticide chemist, we can argue that he has picked both a spouse and a boss with whom it is not possible to be angry despite their unreasonable behaviour. On this argument, his spouse and boss were people with whom others would also have found it difficult to become angry. It is thus not this difficulty, but rather the pesticide chemist's choice of these people as his spouse and boss, that reflects the effect of his childhood relationship with his father on his adult life and thus establishes the primary importance of that relationship.

But this cannot be a complete answer to the suggestion that it may simply be the pesticide chemist's behaviour as a child that produced the difficulties in his childhood relationship with his father, just as his present behaviour is supposed to have produced the difficulties in his adult relationships with his spouse and boss. The theme of anger's not being expressed is also supposed to appear in the patient's relationship with his therapist, according to Malan's triangle of person, and the selection of the therapist is a decision over which the patient will presumably have exercised little or no choice. If Malan's triangle of person is accepted, therefore, it seems that the theme of anger's not being expressed in the pesticide chemist's various relationships is unlikely to relate only to the fact that people with whom he chooses to interact are of a certain type.

Although a full discussion of the point is beyond the scope of the present account, it is worth noting here that some psychodynamic formulations seem as if they probably *overstate* the contribution a person makes as a child to the nature of his or her relationships with adults – that is, these formulations make precisely the opposite error to that which it has been argued Malan makes as regards the pesticide chemist.

Perhaps there are other features of this case that might suggest the pesticide chemist's relationship with his father to be of primary importance. For example, the good intentions with which his father was absent from home – attempting to earn money for his family – might have made it genuinely inappropriate to be angry with him. Despite this, it might be suggested, his son was angry with him, and this is what produced the pesticide chemist's difficulties in expressing anger even when it is appropriate in adult life. According to this position, then, it is not merely the similarities between the pesticide chemist's childhood relationship with his father on the one hand, and his adult relationships on the other, that justify Malan's assigning the former its primary importance. As mentioned in Section 5.4.3, Malan puts forward this view in his discussion. Alternatively or additionally, it might have been that the pesticide chemist was *actively encouraged* as a child not to express his feelings.

The evidence in favour of these possibilities does not seem to be very strong for the present case. Thus, there is no suggestion at all, in Malan's discussion, of the patient's having been encouraged as a child not to express his feelings. Similarly, it appears as if the behaviour of the pesticide chemist's father was not beyond reproach and that the patient may, indeed, have been quite badly neglected by his father. We are told, for example, that the patient had hardly any home life as a child and, with his father "constantly away, [he] involved himself in activities away from home seven nights a week where in fact he found a substitute father who took him under his wing" (Malan, 1979, p. 105).

5.7 The elimination of body products

There is a further theme that is arguably of importance in characterising Malan's account of the pesticide chemist's difficulties as psychodynamic, although this theme is not very prominent in Malan's discussion of this case. This theme is that of the elimination of body products. In discussing the case of the pesticide chemist, Malan formulates the problem as relating to unexpressed anger, and he stresses the fact that when this patient did finally break down, "his outburst resulted in his *making a mess* "(1979, p. 103, original emphasis); a similar observation was also offered to the patient by his therapist, who suggested that "the feelings that he was so terrified of were strongly aggressive feelings, and that they were to do with the part of him that wanted to let go all his controls and make a mess" (1979, p. 104).

These points refer to a discussion earlier in Malan's chapter, in which he suggests that "it is an empirical fact that in some people [the elimination of body products] takes on a significance apparently out of all proportion to their simple function of expelling unwanted matter from the body" (p. 99). These points also take us back, of course, to Freud's remarks regarding the putative anal-sadistic stage of development and OCD, some comments on which have already been offered (see Section 5.2).

Malan elsewhere suggests that there are at least "two important roots" to this exaggerated importance of body products. The first of these is "some kind of primitive equation between the *inside of the body* and *feelings*, so that elimination of physical matter becomes equated with the expression of feeling" (Malan, 1979, p. 99, original emphasis). The second is that the "struggle of toilet training may come to represent the whole issue of *freedom versus restraint*; and incontinence which results in *making a mess* may become a way of expressing anger and rebellion" (Malan, 1979, p. 99, original emphasis). It is further suggested by Malan that a later struggle over the right to express sexual feelings may reawaken the earlier struggle, and the two may become associated (p. 99). Although he does not say so at this point, Malan elsewhere suggests that this association is facilitated by sexual activity's also involving (at least for men) the elimination of body products; see, for example, Malan's discussion (p. 100) of the difficulties of the maintenance man with nocturnal emissions.

It is clear from his case discussions that although Malan does present the theme that the elimination of body products is linked to OCD, he does not regard this link as *peculiar* to the disorder. For example, the case of the aforementioned maintenance man, which involves a phobic problem, features this theme far more prominently than does that of the pesticide chemist. Malan can thus be arguing only that the elimination of body products takes on a great significance for some people, a proportion of whom happen to be OCD patients.

Malan's position is surely controversial in suggesting that the exaggerated significance of body products relates specifically to the expression of anger. What cannot be denied, however, is that there are some OCD patients for whom contamination with such body products as urine and faeces does have an exaggerated significance. What, then, of Malan's suggestions as to why this should be the case? How well does he explain the disgust with, or fear of, these expelled body products?

Before Malan's explanation of the disgust with, and fear of, expelled body products is discussed, two points should be noted. Firstly, those OCD patients who are strongly inclined to avoid contact with urine and faeces are distinguished from the normal population in degree, rather than in kind, in being so inclined – these products have, in Malan's terms, an exaggerated significance for most people. Secondly, some measure of disgust also seems to be felt by most people toward contact with many other materials that are expelled from inside the body. Thus, this attitude is not restricted to those materials that would have been involved in a person's toilet training or in "the later struggle over the right to express sexual feelings". For example, contact with phlegm, saliva, sweat, vomit, food or drink that has been spat out, and perhaps even ear wax, is usually in some measure aversive for most people (tears seem to be an exception), with this aversion being particularly marked when the saliva, sweat, and so forth is that of another person (the contact between lovers, and between young children and their parents, provide some exceptions to this rule).

As mentioned earlier in this section, Malan suggests that there are two reasons for the exaggerated importance of body products: (1) There is a primitive equation between the inside of the body and feelings, which in turn equates the elimination of physical matter with the expression of feelings; and (2) the struggle of toilet training comes to represent the issue of freedom versus restraint, so that incontinence may become a way of expressing anger and rebellion. The observation that most people seem to feel some measure of disgust toward many materials (other than urine and faeces) expelled from the inside of the body looks as if it may be inconsistent with Malan's second reason. Why should one suppose toilet training, for example, to be of fundamental importance to our understanding of the exaggerated significance of urine and faeces when similar attitudes are found toward other materials that are expelled from the body which have never been involved in such training?

A more parsimonious explanation would apply to the aversion that is felt toward *most* body products, not just toward *some* of them, and Malan's first reason for this aversion appears, in contrast to his second reason, to possess this wider applicability. This explanation, however, meets with other difficulties. The suggested link between the inside of the body and feelings is implausible as an explanation of the aversiveness of body products – it seems that to equate matter from inside the body with feelings would not render such matter aversive in any reliable way, because it is obviously not the case that most or all feelings are aversive. (Even if it were argued here that most of the feelings of some OCD patients are aversive, this still leaves unexplained the milder degree of aversion felt by most people toward body products.) A different explanation is called for, and might perhaps be supplied, contrary to Malan's position, in terms of an innate aversion to body products as possible sources of contamination (see, for example, Gray, 1982, discussed in Sections 3.4 and 3.5).

5.8   Summary and discussion

Some psychodynamic theories of OCD have been briefly outlined, and a case discussion presented by Malan has been examined in some detail. Four features, it has been argued, give this case discussion its psychodynamic character. These four features are the account's reference to unconscious mental processes, its formulation of the patient's concerns as having symbolic significance, its claim that the patient's difficulties may be understood as having occurred in order to serve some purpose for him, and its claim that insight into hidden feelings derived from childhood experience is of fundamental importance to therapeutic outcome. It was argued that if there is anything of a psychodynamic character about the first of these features, this is merely a semantic matter. The other three features are all more substantial, but reasons have been offered for thinking none of them to be important to the understanding of the pesticide chemist's problems.

There are clear links between some of Malan's remarks and Freud's ideas concerning the relationship between the "anal-sadistic" stage and OCD – in particular, the emphasis in Malan's account on the pesticide chemist's hypothesised efforts to control his own anger, and Malan's relating this to the theme of the elimination of body products. Reasons for rejecting Malan's account of the exaggerated importance of body products have been offered. One might suggest, then, that doubts are justified as to the value of the psychodynamic aspects of Malan's account. This is not, of course, to argue that all psychodynamic ideas are of limited value for all cases of OCD; this conclusion is beyond the scope of the present discussion for reasons set out at the start of the chapter. It is suggested that the present discussion has raised a number of difficulties that many psychodynamic approaches to OCD (and indeed to other disorders) will likely often encounter.

It is appropriate to note that the foregoing discussion also shows the psychodynamic aspects of Malan's account to be open to objective criticism, contrary to Popper's (1963, 1972) characterisation of psychodynamic theory. This point is, of course, double edged from the perspective of Malan's discussion – in defending the various psychodynamic aspects of Malan's case discussion from the charge of not being open to objective criticism, it also suggests these various aspects to have been refuted (or at least to have been shown to be implausible in the present case).

None of the foregoing implies that Malan's discussion fails in all respects to illuminate the difficulties of the pesticide chemist. They also do not imply that this discussion would be entirely unhelpful in explaining the difficulties of some other OCD patients. Some of Malan's remarks made in connection with the triangle of conflict for the pesticide chemist seem as if they may be of value – in particular, his suggestions that the pesticide chemist's unassertive behaviour contributed to the production of the patient's problems and that "constructive assertion" has helped to relieve these problems (see Chapter 8). It is only being suggested here that, in making no reference to symbolisation, defence mechanisms and the like, these suggestions concerning anger and unassertive behaviour do not contribute to the specifically psychodynamic character of Malan's account. This claim is largely a semantic matter, merely a question of stipulating what may and what may not be termed psychodynamic; the suggested justification for this stipulation is that accounts from quite other perspectives offer very similar suggestions regarding the role of unassertive behavior in OCD and other patients (for example, see Section 4.7.3 and Chapter 8). It is perhaps more important to note that some psychodynamic accounts – including Malan's case discussion and Freud's remarks on anal-sadism and OCD – may be drawing attention to an important element in at least some cases of OCD by pointing out the possible role played by unexpressed anger. This claim will be examined further in Chapter 8.

6 Cognitive style/deficit approaches to OCD

6.1 Reed's account

6.1.1 Reed's hypothesis of the central problem

A number of authors (for example, Beech and Perigault, 1974; Beech and Liddell, 1974; Carr, 1974; Volans, 1974, 1976; Reed, 1985, 1991) have suggested that a generalised cognitive style or deficit in OCD sufferers may be responsible for the occurrence of OCD symptoms. Reed's ideas represent the most fully worked out contribution from this school. He advances what he terms a "cognitive-structural approach" (Reed, 1985) to explain both the obsessional personality (and personality disorder) and OCD. In what follows, the term *obsessional* will be used generically, as it is by Reed, to cover OCD, the obsessional personality/personality disorder, and the person who exhibits either of these. Unlike many of the approaches discussed in other chapters of this book, Reed's account has not been subject to widespread critical discussion; particularly detailed consideration of this account is therefore offered here.

What, then, is the central problem in obsessional disorders, according to Reed? His attempts to answer this question in just a few words tend to be a little cryptic. For example, he suggests that obsessional traits and symptoms reflect difficulties in "spontaneous categorizing and integration" (1985, p. 220) leading to attempts to compensate for these difficulties by "the artificial over-structuring of input, of fields of awareness, of tasks and situations" (p. 220); there is, he argues, a "maladaptive over-defining of categories and boundaries" (1969b, p. 787). Reed states that the central phenomenon of these disorders "may thus be seen as a striving towards boundary fixing or the setting of limits in the cognitive/perceptual modalities" (1985, p. 220).

What all this amounts to may perhaps be made a little clearer by reflecting upon what Reed presents as one example of laboratory-based confirmation of his account. Reed (1969b) presented subjects with blocks of various shapes, sizes and colours and asked them to form classes of these blocks in any way they thought sensible – that is, to choose for themselves the features on the basis of which the blocks were to be classified.

Reed correctly predicted that his obsessional group (all of whom were diagnosed as suffering from obsessional personality disorder) would tend to assign fewer blocks to each of the classes they formed than would controls and therefore would require more classes to complete this task. Reed suggested that this was because his obsessional subjects, in contrast to his controls, would tend to experience doubts as to the appropriate ordering of the categorisable features of the blocks in terms of their task relevance and importance. Reed suggested that his obsessional subjects, in contrast to controls, found it more difficult to order these features "hierarchically", tending to experience doubts as to whether remote or unlikely differences between blocks were as important as obvious similarities. This rendered it more difficult for them to be certain that any two (or more) blocks were sufficiently similar to be classified together.

Consider an example. Suppose that among the blocks presented to subjects were two red cubes of slightly different sizes and a blue pyramid. Reed's suggestion is that obsessional subjects would be more likely than controls to feel uncertain that the similarities between the cubes in terms of their shape and colour were more important than their slight difference in size for the purposes of classification on this task. This renders it both more difficult for these subjects to make a spontaneous decision as to how to classify these blocks, and less likely that they will classify them in the most straightforward way – in this case, in terms of colour and shape, thus placing the red cubes together and separate from the blue pyramid. It is also more likely that, to classify the blocks, they will need more categories than controls will. Thus, Reed suggests that obsessionals, in contrast to controls, fail to discard "torturous and arbitrary" complicating features (minor differences in size, in the present case) that controls consider to be of little importance to the task, and so these complicating features are also more likely to turn up among the criteria chosen by obsessionals to classify the blocks. Thus, the obsessionals in the given example would be more likely, relative to controls, to classify the two cubes separately, as well to keep them both separate from the blue pyramid.

Using the terms of Reed's hypothesis, one can say that the difficulties of obsessionals in "spontaneous categorizing and integration" are, in the case of the block-sorting task, the uncertainties as to the ordering of the categorisable features of the blocks according to their relevance and importance. Obsessionals' "artificial over-structuring" of the task, their "maladaptive over-defining of categories and boundaries", is their tendency to include among the criteria employed in forming their classes "remote and unlikely" features of the blocks and, thus, to form a larger number of classes. This inclusion of such features is also an example of the obsessionals' "striving towards boundary fixing or the setting of limits" (1985, p. 220).

Reed uses this task to examine what his obsessional subjects would do in what he describes as an "inductive situation" – that is, where the task requirement is "to induce concepts or classes given an array of class members (rather than deduce which members belong to a given class)" (1969b, p. 787). Reed also reports a confirmation of his hypothesis with a "deductive task" (1969a), but his position is that obsessionals will face "most difficulty in open-ended tasks requiring an intuitive approach and/or *inductive* reasoning" (1985, p. 194, original emphasis). He presents an experimental confirmation of this suggestion, once again using patients diagnosed as suffering from obsessional personality disorder

(1977b). It seems, then, that it is the performance of obsessionals on Reed's inductive classificatory task to which we should turn for what Reed deems to be the best analogue of the difficulties experienced by obsessional patients.

Consider, then, Reed's approach as applied, for example, to compulsive handwashing. The nonobsessional subject experiences no difficulty in feeling satisfied that his hands have been properly or sufficiently washed – in particular, minor details regarding the exact manner in which his handwashing has been performed, or the precise feel of his hands after washing them, and so on, do not determine whether or not satisfaction is achieved. This is in contrast, Reed suggests, to the compulsive handwasher (1985, p. 165): a feeling of doubts regarding such details as these will prevent his feeling satisfied that the task has been properly done. These doubts, then, are the failure of the compulsive handwasher to structure or integrate this task spontaneously. Ritualistic handwashing, in which a detailed specification is made as to exactly how this task is to be carried out, is the attempt of the handwasher to compensate for his difficulty in spontaneously structuring or integrating the task by artificially overstructuring it.

Reed claims that this difficulty with spontaneous structuring and artificial overstructuring is the "central psychological phenomenon" (1985, p. 117) of all the "classical symptoms" of OCD – although remarks he makes concerning redintegration elsewhere in his discussion suggest that he would only wish to defend a somewhat qualified version of this thesis (see Section 6.1.2).

Reed also presents (1985, Chapter 5) a discussion of thirty-three traits that are most commonly accepted as being among the constituents of the obsessional personality and personality disorder, and he argues that these, too, are susceptible to analysis in terms of his hypothesis.

Reed's position might appear from the foregoing to be tautological. What we mean – or at least one of the things we can mean – by saying that someone is obsessional about his performance of any task is that, as compared with others, he pays undue attention to the details of that task. Reed's hypothesis is in essence this claim that details are noticed more by obsessionals, and the hypothesis, it might be argued, therefore fails to make any empirical claim at all.

This objection to Reed's position as tautological can be rejected. Reed is explicit as regards two points to which his analysis gives rise, both of which are substantial – and indeed highly controversial – empirical claims.

6.1.1.1 *Reed's first controversial empirical claim*

Reed suggests that the thinking style detailed in his hypothesis is the *primary dysfunction* in – the root of – obsessional disorders. To return to the handwashing example to illustrate this, Reed's position is that the attention to detail described is not the result of any emotional problem, such as a greater-than-normal fear of germs or disgust at dirt. The distress reported, he suggests, is rather an *effect* of the sufferer's way of performing the task – an effect of his difficulty in feeling satisfied that the task has been adequately performed. Reed thus suggests that the distress involved in these disorders stems not from *that which* the sufferer thinks about, but rather from his *manner of thinking* about it; not from that which the sufferer does, but rather from his manner of doing it (Jakes, 1987). Putting this rather differently, Reed argues that the problems "of obsessionals concern the *form* [of experience] rather than [its] *content*" (1991, p. 88, emphasis added; see Section 4.9.3.1 for an interpretation of some of Pitman's [1987b] remarks that is similar to this view).

Reed believes, consistent with this account, that the major mood disturbance in obsessional disorders is not anxiety, and he argues that both behavioural and psychoanalytic theorists place too much emphasis upon this emotion in their explanations of obsessional disorders. He suggests (1985, p. 137) that "there appears to be no convincing evidence that anxiety plays a significant role in obsessional disorder" and argues that, where anxiety does occur, "it is usually related to long term apprehension, rather than the immediate experience"; that is, the handwasher's anxiety will concern such matters as the possibility of his never getting over his problem, rather than dirt or germs. Reed lays stress upon there being other kinds of mood disturbances that are frequently reported by obsessionals (such as depression, anger and frustration), these being distress of a type, he suggests, that may be readily explained consistently with his hypothesis as being the result of the sufferer's having difficulties in spontaneously structuring the tasks that provoke these mood disturbances.

Reed stresses (1968, pp. 288–9) that patients often report their decision difficulties not "to bear any direct relation to the importance or emotionally-chargedness" of the situation in which the difficulties arise, such difficulties often concerning details the patients themselves recognise to be "prosaic, trivial and unthreatening" (1991, p. 80). Reed provides examples of patients whose greatest agonies of doubt concern whether or not to tie their shoelaces or whether or not to get up out of a chair. Another example would be that of patients' having to place a book on a table so that its edges are parallel to those of the table, despite no outcome of any significance being feared should this not be done (see Section 1.3.4.6). Reed argues that such phenomena support his account of obsessional disorders and suggests that "content approaches [he includes behavioural and psychoanalytic approaches, as well as most other kinds, in this category] are less likely to be productive and generalisable than approaches that aim to uncover the form or structure of obsessional thinking in general" (1991, pp. 80–1).

6.1.1.2 Reed's second controversial empirical claim

Equally central to Reed's position is his suggestion that the thinking style detailed in his hypothesis is *general* to the sufferer's functioning – that it is part of the sufferer's personality structure – rather than being specific to particular symptom areas. A close relationship between the obsessional personality (and personality disorder) and OCD is therefore proposed, the symptoms of OCD being, according to Reed's account, "simply pathological extensions" (1985, p. 117) of the traits of the obsessional personality and personality disorder. Although Reed can, therefore, concede that symptoms other than those classifiable as OCD may be experienced by someone with an obsessional personality, he is committed to the view that OCD symptoms cannot emerge in the *absence* of this obsessional personality (or even, perhaps, in the absence of the personality disorder).

6.1.2 Reed on therapeutic approaches

In the light of his analysis, Reed suggests that it is the central task of interventions with obsessional disorders to change the patient's style of cognitive functioning. Although Reed suggests a number of treatment techniques designed to achieve this (1985, pp. 225–6), he unfortunately presents no data showing how effective these techniques are.

In addition to suggesting these techniques, Reed notes "some popular therapeutic measures which, in the light of the present theory, are either contra-indicated or at least time-wasting" (1985, p. 221). Of interest is his inclusion of assertiveness training and exposure with response prevention among such therapeutic measures. Reed suggests that assertiveness training does not seem to be "even remotely relevant to obsessional disorder" (1985, p. 222), obsessional patients tending to be opinionated and overassertive. (This supposed feature of people with obsessional disorders presumably follows, according to Reed, from their overstructuring approach.)

Regarding exposure with response prevention, Reed argues that the achievements of this approach have been confined to the reduction of compulsive behaviour, with little or no progress having been made with the remediation of obsessions (1985, p. 208); Reed appears to hold that this supposed outcome is pretty much what his account would predict for behavioural approaches.

Reed also objects to the use of cognitive therapy with obsessionals, although here the basis of his objection is what Reed takes to be the *defining criteria* of the symptoms of OCD. He points out that Beck's therapeutic techniques, for example, involve encouraging the patient who is suffering from depression or anxiety to gain insight into the irrationality of the thinking that is postulated by this therapeutic approach to be the primary difficulty in these mood disturbances. This approach is inappropriate for obsessional disorders, Reed argues (1985, p. 213), because by definition these patients already have insight into the thoughts that preoccupy them.

6.1.3 The redintegration hypothesis

Reed (1977a, 1985) supplements his account with the suggestion that some obsessional symptoms reflect the "faulty redintegration" of memories, this supposedly resulting from the patient's hypothesised problems in structuring experience.

Why does Reed make this suggestion, and what exactly does it mean? Reed (1977a, p. 178) correctly points out that his original hypothesis "makes no direct presumption about mnemonic processes". Thus, his original hypothesis attempts to explain why a patient may feel unsure that, for example, some act has been properly performed or some thought adequately considered, but it makes no attempt to explain why a patient should not feel sure that he has or has not even attempted to perform some act. The obsessional patient, that is, is hypothesised by Reed to have difficulties in spontaneously organising the details of his performance, not in recollecting these details themselves.

Yet some symptoms, Reed points out, do appear to involve difficulties in recollection that are of this kind. Reed himself, indeed, suggests that "perhaps the most central feature of obsessional disorders seems to involve pathologically *faulty* memory" (1977a, p. 177, original emphasis), and he suggests that the "doubts and indecision...manifested in compulsive checking...are often of the 'Did I or Didn't I?' variety" (1977a, p. 177). These patients, that is, sometimes do doubt whether they have carried out certain actions *at all*, rather than doubt only whether these actions have been performed properly; this point is especially clear in those cases where the patient fears that he may have performed some horrific act, such as strangling an elderly next door neighbour. The doubt here could evidently not be, "Have I strangled this elderly person *properly*?" – rather, it would be, "Have I done this terrible thing at all?"

Reed thus raises a difficulty for his account in its original form that he attempts to solve by introducing the notion of the "faulty redintegration of memories". Memories that exhibit this feature have an "attenuation of the personalised element", Reed explains (1985, p. 154) – the person recalls what he has done or what has happened to him, but in a manner such that it is as if *he* has not done these things or had these things happen to *him*.

Reed suggests that the memory difficulties of obsessional patients are of this kind. Contrary to what might seem to be the case, Reed tells us, an obsessional does not, for example, check his door because he doubts he has locked it. In defence of this claim, Reed cites the fact that obsessional patients often report that they know their door is locked before checking it. Thus, in explaining the checker's need to repeat his action, Reed says that "something paradoxical about compulsive checking is indicated. For the compulsive checker often reports that he knows that the door is locked *before* he checks....The question seems to have already been answered...[yet] the compulsive checker's doubts have not been allayed; his question, then, has not been answered. But, as his check *has*, in fact, answered the question of whether he had locked the back door, his continuing dubiety strongly suggests that *that was not his question*" (1985, p. 151, original emphasis).

What is unsatisfactory about the recollections of these patients and causes them to check is not, according to Reed, "the factual content of their remembering, but *the quality of the remembering itself*" (1985, p. 154, original emphasis). Repetitive checking, Reed suggests, thus "represents an attempt to invoke a satisfactory level of redintegration" (1977, p. 154). He attempts to support this contention with the following extracts from the accounts of his patients: "It's done, I know that – *but I can't see myself doing it*"; "I think I remember all right. But it's blurry somehow – *as though I'm not there*"; "I know they are O.K. When I think back I can see them in my head. The trouble is that I can't be sure that *it was me seeing them before...*" (1985, p. 153, original emphasis).

Attempting to link this point to his central hypothesis, Reed suggests, following Bartlett (1932), that this "personalized flavour of reminiscence must reflect...the level and scope of schematization of the original experience" (Reed, 1985, p. 197). "If the anankast [that is, the obsessional] suffers impairment in the organization and integration of experience, this would imply some attenuation in schematization (including the personal element)", Reed argues (1977a, p. 178).

Objections to this "faulty redintegration" analysis will be considered later. Attempting for the moment to clarify what exactly is being argued, consider this analysis a little more closely. Reed appears to be arguing that the repeated actions that result from putative difficulties in redintegration do not involve the patient's adjusting minor details of each successive action and similarly do not involve the patient's worrying that the details of the performance of these actions have been inadequate, in contrast to the handwashing example discussed in Section 6.1.1. The patient's doubt simply concerns the lack of a "subjective flavour" to his recall, according to Reed, and the act is repeated in an attempt to establish such a flavour. (The patient is evidently also supposed by Reed to be unaware that the absence of this subjective flavour is in fact caused by his poor spontaneous structuring; otherwise, the patient presumably *would* attempt to adjust minor details of his actions in an attempt to improve the structuring, and thus [on Reed's view] his redintegration, of those actions.)

All of the examples Reed discusses in terms of redintegration relate to checking and rumination. Furthermore, the discussion Reed offers of a case of handwashing (1985, p. 166) seems very clearly to be an account of this phenomenon in terms of his original hypothesis unsupplemented by the notion of redintegration. Are these examples, then, considered by Reed to be *typical*? Is Reed's redintegration explanation being applied to checking and rumination, but not to cleaning? The author has been unable to find a discussion of these points in Reed's work, but it does seem as if Reed's theoretical position would make this exclusion of cleaning problems difficult to sustain. The problems in redintegration, after all, are supposed to result from difficulties in spontaneously categorising, so Reed would presumably expect most or all obsessionals to exhibit both types of problem and to tend to do so in the same situations and on the same tasks. But clarification of Reed's position regarding his redintegration hypothesis is rendered rather difficult by his seeming failure to incorporate this hypothesis into summaries of his position. Thus, in stating the essence of his theory, Reed suggests (1985, p. 221) that checking and ruminations – the two phenomena he had previously discussed in terms of poor redintegration (1985, pp. 197–8) – may be seen as reflecting a failure in "terminating response", coupled with uncertainty in categorical limit attribution ("Is it finished?"). This applies to inner reasoning ("Has everything been considered?"), to mnemonic brooding ("Are my recollections sufficient and correct?"), and to the consideration of activities ("Did I do it properly?"). The questions are insoluble, because such qualifiers as "finished", "sufficiently", "satisfactorily" and "properly", cannot be defined in any ultimate and fixed manner. (Reed, 1985, p. 221)

The notion of redintegration appears to have been entirely overlooked here.

6.2 Objections to the redintegration hypothesis

There are a number of objections that apply specifically to the redintegration supplement, instead of to Reed's account as a whole. Four of these objections will be discussed. Firstly, the quotes from patients by which Reed tries to support his reintegration hypothesis feature such comments as, "...but I can't see myself doing it", or "It's as though I'm not there", made as these people describe their attempts to recall previous checks they have carried out. It is surely unclear that such locutions as these amount to more than mere expressions of doubt as to whether or not these checks have been made. There is, furthermore, no claim on Reed's part that these choices of words are *systematically* used by obsessionals. These extracts are merely examples that have been quoted *precisely because* of the particular choice of words involved. It seems likely that checkers often express their doubts in quite other ways, and so Reed is probably placing too much stress on the particular terms used by the patients he quotes.

Secondly, the fact that the obsessional will often say that she knows, for example, that her door is locked before checking it, is used by Reed (1985, p. 151) to support his claim that the checking does not concern the state of the door at all but rather concerns the quality of the patient's memories. But there may be difficulties with this argument, because Reed is prepared to recognise that in cases of obsessional difficulties not involving redintegration at all, the patient will still report insight of this kind; indeed, he argues elsewhere (1985, pp. 4–5) that this feature must, *by definition*, be present in *every* case of OCD (see Section 1.2.2), whereas he evidently believes that the redintegration hypothesis can be applied to only some kinds of obsessional problem.

Thirdly, Reed takes as his starting point in introducing the notion of reintegration the "Did I or didn't I?" *doubts* of obsessional checkers and ruminators. But can this account explain why doubts are reported at all by these patients? On this "'faulty redintegration" hypothesis, the checker has no doubts as to what has occurred, she simply has a memory that lacks a given property – its subjective flavour – and the patient's repeated actions are supposed to be an attempt to add this property. So where does the patient come by her *doubt*, according to Reed?

One reply that Reed might have made is that the lack of a subjective flavour to the patient's recall in some way leads her to doubt whether or not the remembered event or action has taken place. But Reed could clearly make this reply only by sacrificing the claim, emphasised in presenting his redintegration supplement, that the patient's doubts and repeated actions are not related to checking the state of the door at all.

Fourthly, Reed's redintegration hypothesis fails to explain all of the phenomena that it was introduced to deal with. These include not only cases where patients repeat actions that they have already performed, but also cases where they fear that they *may* have performed some action that has in fact *not* been performed, such as some violent behaviour. How can such cases be explained in terms of the level of redintegration of the original experience, when there has been no original experience? If Reed's redintegration account can be extended to explain these cases, he does not suggest how this should be done.

6.3   A motivational problem for Reed's account

As we have seen, Reed's account attempts to explain why an obsessional patient might find it difficult to feel certain that, for example, his hands have been properly cleaned. Yet if the patient were entirely indifferent as to whether or not his hands were so cleaned, there would be no problem for him, however difficult it was for him to feel certain that this state had been achieved.

What thus appears to be taken for granted by Reed's account is that such a patient *needs* to feel certain that his hands have been properly washed. This raises an important problem for Reed's account, because the patient's behaviour suggests that his problem is not just a matter of his having more difficulty feeling certain that actions have been properly carried out. A *greater intolerance* of such feelings of uncertainty is additionally, or instead, implied. The compulsive handwasher, for example, appears to be less able than others to bear the possibility that his hands may be contaminated; it *matters* more to him that they are not. And Reed's account appears to be silent as to why this should be so. Though most noncompulsive washers would no doubt prefer their hands to be properly clean – at least at mealtimes and the like – they will, in the ordinary course of things, be able to tolerate the thought that their hands are not properly clean. If, for example, time is short or the noncompulsive handwasher finds himself in a frame of mind such that he simply cannot be bothered to visit the bathroom, he will be able to bear not merely the uncertainty that his hands may not be properly washed, but indeed the certainty that they are not. We may conclude that the inability to determine whether or not tasks such as handwashing have been properly carried out cannot be the only factor that distinguishes obsessional patients from others. This difficulty – its mattering more to obsessional patients that, for example, their hands have been properly cleaned – will be referred to as the *motivational problem* in what follows. (The same difficulty was introduced for part of Pitman's [1987a] account in Section 4.9.3.1.)

The motivational problem also arises as regards those cases (cited by Reed as especially favouring his hypothesis) in which obsessional patients are distressed by concerns that they themselves recognise to be trivial and prosaic. Consider the example presented earlier of having to place a book on a table so that it is perfectly parallel to the table edges, despite no outcome of any significance being feared by the patient should she fail to do this. Although the patient in this example may describe the situation of the book's not being parallel with the table edges as trivial, she is nonetheless unable to tolerate the book's being placed in any manner other than parallel. This, then, surely distinguishes her from a nonobsessional person – such a person will simply not care whether or not the book has been placed parallel to the table's edges. The obsessional does not, therefore, differ from others only (if indeed at all) in terms of how precisely she judges whether or not the two edges are parallel. The motivational problem for Reed's account therefore arises – a *greater intolerance* of the book's not being parallel to the table edges is implied, and Reed's account provides no explanation of this. (The motivational problem may also be raised against Reed's redintegration account. Even if it were true that, for example, a checker's recall of her action lacks a subjective flavour, why should this matter to the patient? Why, on Reed's account, is this quality so important to the checker that it is worth her repeating her actions many times in an attempt to establish it? Reed's redintegration hypothesis evidently just *assumes* that, from the patient's point of view, it is worth her repeating her action in order to establish this.)

The following two replies to the motivational problem might be suggested in defence of Reed's account. Firstly, not *all* nonobsessional patients will be able to tolerate the thought that, for example, their hands have not been properly washed. Obsessionality is a continuum, and it might be plausibly argued that some percentage of the population who will never become obsessional patients are nonetheless a sufficient distance along this continuum not to be able to tolerate this thought. According to this argument, what separates the population of obsessional patients from *these* normals could therefore be an inability to determine that, for example, their hands have been properly washed, and it is this inability that could be explained by Reed's account. Cleanliness, on this argument, matters equally to both groups, and it is only the greater inability of the obsessional patients, as explained by Reed's original hypothesis, to determine whether or not things are clean that renders their difficulties more severe.

But this reply only shifts the problem elsewhere, rather than solves it. The inability spontaneously to determine that one's hands are properly clean is being acknowledged by this attempted defence of Reed to be insufficient to distinguish the subclinical group of obsessional normals (along with obsessional patients) from the remainder of the normal population. It is thus conceded by this defence of Reed that cleanliness matters more to the subclinical group (and obsessional patients). Therefore, if Reed's account is to attempt to explain obsessionality per se, rather than merely attempt to explain obsessionality of clinical severity, the motivational problem still stands. His account still says nothing about the distinction being argued by this defence to obtain between this subclinical group and the remainder of the normal population. Besides, it seems unparsimonious to explain the difference between a subclinical group with an above-average degree of obsessionality and the remainder of the normal population entirely in terms of one factor, and the difference between this subclinical group and the clinical obsessional population entirely in terms of another.

A second possible reply that a defender of Reed's position might use is based upon an independent claim of Reed's (1968, p. 290) that compulsive behaviour *increases* discomfort and mood disturbance (see Section 6.10 for a discussion of this claim). This suggestion has also been put forward by other authors, for example Walker (1973), Beech and Perigault (1974), and Beech and Liddell (1974).

Reed's claim might be used to argue that the obsessional patient's greater intolerance of the thought that his hands may not have been properly washed, for example, is in some way secondary to the increasing distress that is being experienced as his compulsive behaviour proceeds. He begins his handwashing, according to this reply, with no greater need to feel certain that his hands have been properly washed than the normal subject does. His inability to establish that his washing has been adequate, however (an inability that is explained by Reed's account), leads to frustration and other mood disturbances that, in turn, lead (perhaps, for example, by increasing the subject's sensitivity to punishment) to an increase in the importance to the patient of his hands' being properly cleaned. This reply would conclude that it is this increase in the importance to the patient of his hands being properly cleaned that leaves the obsessional unable simply to leave his hands feeling that they have not been adequately washed, in contrast to what many normal subjects are able to do.

There are at least two replies to this second defence of Reed's position. Firstly, some authorities (for example, Rachman and Hodgson, 1980) would argue many compulsive rituals to be discomfort *reducing*, contrary to Reed (see Section 6.10). Secondly, this defence of Reed implies that if the obsessional does not even attempt his handwashing ritual, no difficulties would be created for him that are any greater than those encountered by a nonobsessional subject who decided to omit a hand wash, because the obsessional's not even attempting to wash his hands would bypass the increase of mood disturbance that is produced by the obsessional's inability to establish that his hands have been properly cleaned. Against this implication, however, it appears that for many OCD patients, not performing their compulsions provokes a very high degree of discomfort (de Silva, 1988, p. 205), suggesting that this defence must be incorrect for such OCD patients.

A more promising approach might be to postulate a mood disturbance that is not an effect of the postulated thinking style of obsessional patients. This mood disturbance could be suggested to operate *in conjunction with* that thinking style to produce the distress of these patients. Accounts of this type have been put forward by, for example, Beech and Perigault (1974), Beech and Liddell (1974) and Claridge (1985; see Section 3.7 for a discussion of this account). Two points should be noted here. Firstly, these accounts amount to an abandonment of Reed's central claim that the thinking style of the obsessional patient forms the single root of that patient's problems(Section 6.1.1.1). Secondly, the possibility of incorporating Reed's account into an approach such as Claridge's demonstrates that the aforementioned motivational problem cannot in itself render Reed's account unworthy of further research. This account may still be able to provide a *partial* explanation of obsessional disorders, even if the foregoing arguments show that it cannot provide a complete account of them.

6.4 A revision of Reed's account

How might Reed's account be revised to meet the motivational problem discussed earlier? One possible adjustment is the suggestion that it is not in establishing whether or not tasks have been *properly completed* that the patient's thinking style is crucial, but rather in his attempting to establish what are likely to be the *outcomes* of his not properly completing these tasks.

As previously pointed out, Reed suggests that the obsessionals in his block-sorting task tended to experience doubts as to whether remote or unlikely differences between the blocks were as important as obvious similarities. He also argues that this reflects a *general* approach to things by the patient in the "cognitive/perceptual modalities" (1985, p. 220). Could Reed not argue, then, that this style of functioning will also pervade the manner in which the patient *calculates the probable outcomes of the tasks that cause him difficulty* – that is, that the patient will experience doubts as to whether remote and unlikely possible consequences are as probable as outcomes that are in fact much more likely? To give two examples of this hypothesised effect: (1) This revised version of Reed's thesis would suggest that the problems of the obsessional patient with cleaning difficulties result from his having doubts about, or overestimating the likelihood of, serious illness's being contracted from normal household dirt and dust; and (2) this account would similarly suggest that the problems of the obsessional patient with checking difficulties result from his having doubts about, or overestimating the likelihood of, fires or other household disasters' being caused by normal household switches and plugs that have not been turned off or removed.

This adjustment to Reed's account would appear to answer the motivational problem that confronts Reed's thesis. Thus, tasks such as checking and cleaning matter more to obsessionals, according to this adjusted version of Reed's thesis, because these patients are more inclined to think dire consequences likely to follow from such tasks' not being properly completed.

It must be stressed that Reed himself does not appear to put forward anything like this adjusted version of his account – perhaps only because he believes his account to be a sufficient explanation, perhaps because he would actually object to this adjusted version as failing to make good sense of the clinical phenomena.

It should also be noted that this adjusted version of Reed's thesis suggests obsessionals will be more likely than others to be *objectively mistaken* in the calculation of probabilities. This is in contrast to Reed's block-sorting task discussed in Section 6.1.1, where there were only *different styles* of sorting the blocks, no right or wrong way of doing so, and where no objective mistakes in the calculation of probabilities were involved. (It should also be noted that the block-sorting task discussed in Section 6.1.1 therefore stands as a weak analogue, and consequently also a weak confirmation, of this adjusted version of Reed's thesis.) In what follows, the adjustment of Reed's account produced by the introduction of the hypothesised difficulties of obsessionals in handling probabilistic information will be referred to as the *Revised Thesis.*

A rather different attempt to revise Reed's thesis might be mentioned in passing. This attempt suggests that rather than *overestimating the likelihood* of aversive outcomes, obsessionals are instead more inclined simply to care or worry about such outcomes. Thus, on this account, the obsessional does not overestimate the probability of, for example, his house's flooding from a dripping tap, but he does worry more than others about such things happening. This approach would argue that his greater degree of worry is quite consistent with the obsessional's regarding this outcome as extremely unlikely.

This may indeed be a consistent hypothesis; however, stated thus, it cannot be plausibly represented as an adapted version of Reed's thesis. This is because no reference is made to the patient's thinking style in explaining why he worries more than others about the possibilities that he recognises as much as they do to be highly remote. It might be replied that the thinking style involved is precisely the hypothesised tendency to worry more – to have more anxious cognitions, perhaps – about these remote possibilities. But this reply in effect then states that the patient worries more about remote possibilities because his thinking style is such as to worry more about remote possibilities. This tautology obviously contains nothing that suggests that this position has anything at all to do with the account presented by Reed.

There are some important differences between the Revised Thesis and Reed's original account. For example, the Revised Thesis cannot be very readily applied to the trivial and prosaic situations and tasks that provoke compulsive behaviour and that are so emphasised by Reed. At most, it seems that all this position can suggest is that in such cases there must be some highly unlikely feared consequence of not placing a book on a table in a certain way (to return to the earlier example), the probability of which consequence the obsessional has overestimated. That the patients to whom Reed is referring are unable to report such feared consequences would have to be attributed to a lack of insight on their part, according to the Revised Thesis, rather than taken at face value. By the same token, Reed's account is less readily applicable than the Revised Thesis to those cases where fears of highly unlikely outcomes *are* reported.

Distress is not entirely secondary to doubts and compulsive behaviour according to the Revised Thesis – this thesis argues that the discomfort experienced by obsessionals will include the fear which results from the patient's thinking that unfavourable outcomes are likely to occur. Doubts and compulsive behaviour are considered to be, at least in part, the *result* of such discomfort, these doubts and compulsive behavior reflecting the patient's concern that the feared outcome will occur. (See Section 6.5 for some objections to the Revised Thesis's account of such doubts and behaviour.) Would these implications of the Revised Thesis perhaps, then, lead Reed to reject it as inconsistent with what he believes the clinical phenomena to be?

The Revised Thesis may seem very like the position of a theorist such as Carr (1974), who suggests that appraisals of threat are heightened in OCD patients. These patients, Carr argues, make an abnormally high estimate of unfavourable outcomes' occurring in any situation. The Revised Thesis is not, however, equivalent to such a position as this. In a situation of objectively high risk, the Revised Thesis would make a prediction precisely the opposite to that made by Carr's heightened threat appraisal explanation – that is, the Revised Thesis would predict that the obsessional should be inclined, in this situation, to experience doubts as to whether the unlikely chance of a favourable outcome is as probable as the unfavourable outcome that is in fact more likely. The account of some cases of OCD offered by Volans (1974, 1976) may have more in common with the Revised Thesis than Carr's account does.

6.5   Objections to the Revised Thesis

Although it addresses the motivational problem for Reed's account, the Revised Thesis faces difficulties of its own. Why, it might be asked, does the obsessional (according to the Revised Thesis) have problems in convincing himself that his hands are properly clean or that all his light switches are off, and why do these problems lead to repetitive cleaning or checking, accompanied by doubts about the compulsive behaviour, and low levels of discomfort reduction following the carrying out of this behaviour? Can this be a matter only of the perceived likely consequences of failing to carry these tasks out successfully? Would such an account not more readily predict that a very careful performance of the act of cleaning or checking should be enough – just as one no doubt observes cautious, but not endlessly repetitive, behaviour from normals in situations of objective high risk – for example, a surgeon's washing his hands before performing an operation (also see Section 2.5)?

To these questions one might reply that the endless repetition of action by obsessionals, when observed, reflects *the nature of the tasks* with which the patient has difficulties. Thus, according to this reply, the obsessional is struggling to complete tasks that *in objective terms* can only with great difficulty be determined to have been adequately performed. It is this, in conjunction with the obsessional's thinking unfavourable outcomes to be very likely if such tasks are not adequately performed, that produces the patient's profile of repeated, but unsuccessful, attempts to convince himself that these tasks have been so performed.

This reply, however, meets with problems very like those encountered by Rachman and Hodgson's (1980) account of the contrasts between checkers and cleaners (see Section 2.5). When the tasks the obsessional struggles to complete are considered in objective terms, difficulties in being sure as to their successful completion would appear to apply more to the typical cleaning task than to the typical checking task. Thus, from the objective point of view, it would seem comparatively easy to be sure that, for example, all of the plugs in a room have been removed from their sockets – one only has to look in order to see that this is so. This is less true of the task of ensuring that, for example, one's hands are perfectly free from all germs and other invisible contamination. One would then expect, on the basis of these "nature of task demands" points, that it would be cleaners rather than checkers who would tend to show more repetitiveness in their compulsions, more doubts as to how effective their compulsive behaviours have been, and less relief from discomfort from their compulsions. But in fact, as noted in Section 2.5, the situation is precisely *the reverse*.

A combination of the Revised Thesis and the nature of checking tasks cannot, then, be used to explain the low levels of relief, the repetitiveness and the doubting reported by many of the obsessional patients who report checking difficulties. This in turn argues that it is unparsimonious to attempt an explanation of the rarer cases of patients who clean and whose compulsions exhibit these features in terms of a combination of the Revised Thesis and the nature of cleaning task demands, more plausible though this argument seems when considered in isolation from the foregoing discussion of checkers. Besides, cleaning tasks that carry objectively high risks appear not to produce endlessly repetitive behaviour and doubting in normals, as would be predicted by this explanation of the behaviour of obsessional cleaners (see Section 2.5). One may conclude that the revised version of Reed's thesis, though answering the motivational problem, is silent as to the repetitiveness and doubting present in some compulsive behaviour.

In Reed's original account, the patients' difficulties in feeling certain that (some) tasks have been properly completed are addressed, but the obsessional's stronger motivation properly to complete such tasks is not. With the Revised Thesis, the matter is the other way about: Although an attempt is made to give an account of the stronger motivation of obsessionals to complete tasks properly, no explanation is given for their doubts about these tasks' having been properly performed or for their repeated attempts so to perform these tasks.

What then, it might be asked, of simply *combining* these positions, Reed's account being used to explain the obsessional's doubts that tasks have not been properly performed (and the obsessional's resulting repetitive behaviour), the Revised Thesis then being added to this to explain why it is so important to the obsessional that tasks have been so performed?

The main objection to this combined approach may already be clear from the foregoing. Reed himself suggests (see Section 6.1.3) that his original account did not explain all compulsive behaviour, and he acknowledged difficulties for this account specifically as regards the doubting and repetitive behaviour of checkers (and ruminators). The doubting and repetitive behaviour of checkers (and the doubting of ruminators) cannot be explained, therefore, simply by combining

Reed's original account with the Revised Thesis – both of these approaches encounter difficulties in explaining checking behaviour.

There is a further difficulty for the Revised Thesis. A tendency to overestimate the probability that unlikely aversive outcomes will occur can scarcely be *specific* to obsessional disorders. There seem to be no theoretical grounds for supposing that many phobic patients, for example, will be distinguishable from obsessionals on this basis. No doubt many obsessional patients *do* fear outcomes that strike us as unlikely, and indeed in *some* cases it seems to be the very remoteness of the feared possibility that helps to give the patient's anxiety an obsessional, as opposed to a phobic, quality (see Section 1.3.4.4). But many phobic subjects nonetheless appear to fear things as unlikely as, or even more unlikely than, those feared by many obsessionals. Many, if not all, deluded subjects, to take another example, seem similarly inclined to think some events or situations probable or certain to occur (or to have occurred), despite these events' or situations' being in fact highly unlikely (see Sections 1.3.9 and 1.3.10). Many delusions, phobias and obsessional difficulties (no doubt among other psychiatric disorders) are, therefore, indistinguishable from the point of view of the Revised Thesis, which is consequently silent as to why one patient develops one of these disorders whereas another develops one of the others. This point is especially worth noting in connection with the experimental investigations conducted by Volans (1974, 1976), Huq, Garety and Hemsley (1988) and Garety, Hemsley and Wessely (1991). These investigations have examined the handling of probabilistic information by obsessional patients and by deluded patients, and some of these investigations have reported contrasting results from these two groups; the Revised Thesis appears unable to make much sense of these findings. (Reed's account, by contrast, does not appear to encounter any difficulties in distinguishing obsessional disorders from conditions such as delusions and phobic states – his account emphasises features such as the doubting and repetitive behaviour of obsessionals, which distinguish their difficulties from these other conditions; Reed's account appears, if anything, to *overstate* the differences between phobic and obsessional disorders. See Section 6.12.)

What, then, remains of the Revised Thesis after considering all of the foregoing arguments against it? These arguments leave open the possibility that miscalculations of probabilities may help explain various aspects of obsessional disorders. For example, both the compulsive behaviour *and* the fears of a typical cleaner in Rachman and Hodgson's (1980) investigation might be open to such an explanation. (As noted in Section 2.5, Rachman and Hodgson report that the compulsive behaviour of cleaners tends not to exhibit the repetitiveness and high levels of doubt that the Revised Thesis has difficulty explaining.) Fears of remote or unlikely consequences are also reported by many of these patients with cleaning difficulties, which is also consistent with the Revised Thesis.

The fears reported by many checkers also involve a concern with highly remote consequences. Even if the Revised Thesis cannot explain the doubting and repetitiveness that are frequently observed in the compulsive behaviour of such patients, the thesis may still be consistent with the improbable outcomes that concern many patients and thus be able to provide a partial explanation of their difficulties. (Note that it was in effect argued in Section 6.2 that Reed's account is unable to provide even this.)

One can conclude that the Revised Thesis – even when the foregoing criticisms of it have been taken into account – may be worthy of further research, although the thesis in its present form is unable to explain the differences between obsessional difficulties on the one hand, and phobias and delusions on the other.

A number of further important theoretical difficulties confront both Reed's account and the Revised Thesis; these will be reviewed in Section 6.6.

6.6   Further objections to Reed's account

6.6.1   *Obsessional problems not involving doubts, indecision or ritualising*

There are many obsessional difficulties in which the characteristics stressed by Reed's account – doubting, indecision, ritualising and so forth – do not occur at all or are not the only, or primary, feature observed. Consider the following three examples:

(1) DISCRETE OBSESSIONAL THOUGHTS. Instead of a series of doubts or a train of argument, some obsessional patients may be troubled by single thoughts, such as "Christ was a bastard", "I want to sleep with my mother", "I wish my husband were dead". Sometimes discrete visual *images* are reported as the source of distress, these typically involving such contents as "mutilated corpses, decomposing foetuses, my husband involved in a serious motor accident, my parents being violently assaulted" (Rachman and Hodgson, 1980, p. 11).

(2) OBSESSIONAL IMPULSES. Some patients experience the impulse or urge to do something they regard as unacceptable – for example, to perform some harmful or violent act, or to say something of an offensive nature (also see Section 1.3.4.2).

(3) SUPERSTITIOUS THINKING. Such thinking is a prominent feature in some obsessional problems, the patient thinking it necessary, for example, to touch or arrange household objects in a certain way in order to prevent such events as car accidents or other misfortunes, which are in reality entirely unrelated to the behaviour concerned (also see Section 1.3.4.4).

Reed's account seems unable to explain these obsessional difficulties, and the comments he offers as regards both obsessional impulses and discrete obsessional thoughts appear to confirm that this is so. He suggests that obsessional impulses "are often difficult to classify being not so much urges to action as fears, doubts and misgivings *about* urges" (Reed, 1985, p. 17, original emphasis). Surely very few workers in this field would agree with Reed on this point, recognising that the impulse or urge may occur in the absence of such doubts and misgivings, and may itself often be the source of distress for the patient. As regards discrete obsessional thoughts, Reed tells us that these are less common than "older textbooks suggest" (1985, p. 17) and reports as a confirmation of this that only two of the ninety–seven obsessions observed in a sample of fifty of his patients were of this form (1985, p. 18). But Reed's classificatory scheme also includes numerous other categories – for example, an "obsessional fears" category, which accounts for 31% of the obsessions in his sample – and it is not possible to tell from Reed's discussion how many of the obsessions in these other categories might be reclassified as discrete obsessional thoughts.

Reed's account also appears unable to explain why superstitious thinking should occur. Such thinking is clearly *not* a matter of the patient's merely over-structuring a task, although the patterning of behaviour and objects may be observed. The patient is not simply taking greater pains than others to attend to the details of his performance of some ordinary task, as he would in a case of overstructuring. He is, rather, attempting to carry out some entirely abnormal task. The very performance of his action, not merely the manner of this performance, stands in need of explanation.

The Revised Thesis is in a somewhat similar, but not identical, position as to Reed's original account concerning these three types of obsessional difficulties. It, too, can offer no account of obsessional impulses and is similarly silent regarding at least most cases of discrete obsessional thoughts. It is, however, able to make better sense of symptoms involving superstitious thinking than is Reed's original account. The Revised Thesis was primarily introduced, after all, to explain obsessional symptoms where the feared outcome reported was of a highly unlikely nature. It seems that this thesis can deal with superstitious thinking as an instance, or extension, of such fears.

6.6.2 *Obsessional problems that do involve doubts and indecision*

Problems also confront Reed's account for many cases in which the doubts and indecision stressed by this account are observed. Firstly, as pointed out in criticisms of cognitive style/deficit accounts in general (for example, Rachman and Hodgson, 1980; Emmelkamp, 1982), the difficulties of obsessional patients often involve doubts that concern only a few tasks or situations – or even only one task or situation – that the patients must deal with. Why are multiple doubts concerning an endless variety of tasks and situations not observed, as would be predicted by Reed's account?

Reed's reply here is straightforward. He says that it is a "significant fact that severe obsessionals seldom suffer from a single, discrete obsession" (1985,

p. 24). It is therefore "puzzling" to Reed (1985, p. 25) that Rachman and Hodgson (1980) report 73% of their patients to have a single, predominating obsession. Also, Reed (1985, p. 25) interprets the data from a study by Akhtar et al. (1975) as showing that 51% of the patients had multiple obsessions (thus leaving 49% of the sample *without* multiple obsessions). These figures do not seem to support the assertion that severe obsessionals seldom suffer from a single obsession. Reed hints as to how he might tackle this point: "Obsessional people are often embarrassed about their experiences, and when forced to seek help they typically report only the most incapacitating of their problems" (1985, p. 24). Clearly, there may well be something in this point, but it risks degenerating into the unfalsifiable claim that any patient who reports only a single obsession would tell us of further obsessions if only he were less embarrassed or more forthcoming. Therefore, in the absence of positive evidence that more of the patients of the kind questioned by Rachman and Hodgson (1980) and Akhtar et al. (1975) would have reported multiple obsessions in other circumstances, we must conclude that many obsessionals probably do experience only single, or just a few, obsessions and that Reed's account makes poor sense of this observation.

A somewhat related point is that the *content* of many obsessions appears to be highly selective, with certain themes – contamination, sex, violence – featuring far more frequently than would be expected by chance alone (Akhtar et al., 1975; also see Sections 2.2, 3.4, 3.5 and 4.5.5).

How might Reed, then, explain why obsessions should tend to concern some themes much more often than others, and/or why many patients do not suffer from multiple obsessions? As mentioned earlier (Section 6.1.1), he does suggest that most difficulty will be encountered by obsessionals when performing tasks requiring "an intuitive approach and/or inductive reasoning" (1985, p. 194), but it seems clear that this suggestion is not sufficiently specific to explain either the highly selective nature of the content of many obsessions or those patients who report only one obsession or just a few obsessions.

In his very last contribution to the topic of obsessional disorders, Reed makes a further suggestion – that "the personal significance of the item under consideration...will load the cognitive functioning affectively, *and may thus accentuate its operating characteristics*" (1991, p. 79, emphasis added). In the same chapter he similarly suggests that "obsessional decision making may be made even more difficult when the material to be sorted is of a disturbing nature. The question invites empirical examination" (p. 83) (also see Persons and Foa's 1984 findings, and Jakes, 1992, Chapter 5). Indeed, in the conclusion of the same discussion, Reed (1991, p. 96) even argues that "whether this [cognitive] style operates in all mental activities or whether it emerges only in the context of threatening events is as yet unresolved". This last remark, however, is out of step with all of Reed's other statements on this topic (even some in this last discussion) – including, for example, those just quoted as well as his further comment that "by definition, the cognitive style is employed in processing the material, the material does not engender the style. Contents are limitless, but the form is invariant" (pp. 79–80). And to concede that the patient's dysfunctional cognitive style might arise only when he is dealing with disturbing material is to take up a position such as Claridge's (1985; see Section 3.7.2), which, as noted earlier (Section 6.3), abandons, rather than qualifies, Reed's central claim that the thinking style of obsessional patients is the heart of their distress. And so long as this claim is insisted upon (even if one does allow that contents may exercise some influence over form), it seems that one cannot very readily explain either the selectivity of the contents of obsessions or the patients who suffer from just one obsession or a few obsessions. Reed's account, therefore, is more plausible as regards those patients who suffer from an obsessional personality disorder or from multiple obsessions with numerous idiosyncratic contents. It must at least be supplemented if it is to accommodate the selectivity of the contents of obsessions and the fact that many patients appear only to suffer from one obsession or only a few obsessions.

How, then, might Reed's account be so supplemented? One possibility is as follows. Rachman and de Silva's (1978) findings indicate that "normal obsessions", which have contents very similar to the abnormal obsessions suffered by patients, are common in the experience of many people. This could be used to help explain why the abnormal obsessions experienced by patients tend to have the contents they do. These contents, according to this argument, can be explained in the same terms as those in which the contents of normal obsessions are explained, these terms being assumed to be independent of Reed's account. The postulated thinking style of obsessional patients could then be introduced to explain why the patient is so incapacitated when he tries to settle such doubts as, for example, whether or not he has harmed somebody while walking down the street. It might be similarly postulated that the mechanisms responsible for the production of obsessions with these contents also determine the number of obsessions by which the person is troubled and thus help explain those cases where only one obsession is, or just a few obsessions are, experienced.

There are problems for this supplemented version of Reed's account. Firstly, an explanation will still need to be provided as to why the thinking style of these patients operates only on thoughts with such contents, and not (or at least not to the same extent) on other thoughts. Unless some account of this can be provided, the problems of single, predominating obsessions, and of the selectivity of content, reemerge. Secondly, it would appear that the doubting experienced by patients who suffer such obsessions as, "Have I harmed someone as I walked down the street?" is often not of the kind required by Reed's account; that is, the doubting of these patients does not involve a string of various "What if?" questions in which numerous remotely possible ways in which this could have occurred are considered. (That many such doubts appear *not* to take this form is what led Reed himself to introduce the redintegration hypothesis – see Section 6.1.3.) Thirdly, this supplemented version of Reed's thesis lacks parsimony. Whatever the manner in which this account attempts to explain the normal obsessions experienced by many people, it is essential to the account that this explanation cannot make reference to the cognitive style postulated by Reed, which the account does use to explain the difference between normal and abnormal obsessions (otherwise the difficulties concerning selectivity and single obsessions would be introduced). A more parsimonious account, then, would not seek to explain normal obsessions in one way, and the difference between these and abnormal obsessions in quite another. A similar difficulty concerning a lack of parsimony was raised for another supplemented version of Reed's account (discussed in Section 6.3) and for Salkovskis's account of OCD (see Section 2.8; also see Jakes, 1989b.) The supplemented version of Reed's thesis under consideration here, like that discussed in Section 6.3, fails to explain obsessionality per se, attempting instead merely to explain only obsessionality of clinical severity.

6.7   Comments on Reed's remarks regarding therapeutic approaches

Numerous points need to be made regarding Reed's comments on the remediation of obsessional disorders (see Section 6.1.2). Firstly, Reed claims that the achievements of behaviour therapy have been confined to the reduction of compulsive behaviours, with little or no progress having been made with the obsessional experiences that provoke such behaviour. In Reed's view, the patient's style of cognitive functioning would have to be changed in order to reduce or eliminate the patient's obsessional experiences. Reed believes, as discussed earlier, that this can be achieved by running patients through cognitive exercises, including tasks in which the "stress is placed upon speed of performance rather than accuracy" – the crucial ingredient to the intervention, in Reed's view (Reed, 1985, p. 225). Yet in exposure with response prevention, it is precisely this kind of approach that is often adopted, but with respect to the activities that provoke the patient's major difficulties, rather than to artificially constructed tasks (which, on Reed's view, can surely make exposure with response prevention only more powerful – if it makes any difference at all). A patient on a programme of exposure with response prevention may be asked, for example, to complete his cleaning and checking tasks much more quickly than he has done hitherto – that is, with the stress being placed upon the speed of performance, not its accuracy. Why, then, given Reed's own therapeutic recommendations, should Reed believe that this will have no impact on the patient's obsessional experience – his fears, doubts, urges to clean or check, and so forth – and will alter only the compulsive behaviours provoked by such experiences?

Reed may misrepresent the outcome data from behaviour therapy with obsessionals. It *is* true that so far behaviour therapists have had limited success with obsessional difficulties involving *only* covert phenomena (see Section 2.6). But where covert phenomena, such as doubts, fears, urges and so on, do provoke compulsions, these therapists (for example, Rachman and Hodgson, 1980) argue that in many cases, exposure with response prevention has a considerable impact on both the patient's obsessions and his compulsions, and achieves, according to these therapists, considerable success with both phenomena (see Section 2.4).

Secondly, Reed's suggestion that assertiveness training is misconceived with obsessionals because such patients are opinionated and overassertive must be challenged. Janet (1903), for example, remarks upon the unassertive nature of many of his obsessional patients (see Section 4.4). As noted earlier (Section 4.5.2), Lewis (1936, p. 328) postulates *two* types of obsessional personality, "the one obstinate, morose, irritable, the other vacillating, uncertain of himself, submissive". It seems clear that only the former group corresponds to Reed's description, the latter presenting precisely the *opposite* profile. Ingram (1961, discussed by Rachman and Hodgson, 1980) claims that only just under half of his obsessional patients could be described in one or the other of these ways, but among those who could be so classified, he found twice as many of the submissive type of patient as of the obstinate/morose type. Indeed, elsewhere in his discussion, Reed himself (1985, p. 200) notes (as a paradox) that obsessionals are "inflexible and un-shifting [yet] they are also reported to be unassertive and vacillating". Some authors also argue that there is empirical evidence against Reed's claim that assertiveness training cannot help obsessionals (Emmelkamp and van der Heyden, 1980). This evidence, along with some remarks as to its implications for our understanding of obsessional disorders, is discussed elsewhere (see Section 4.7.3 and Chapter 8).

Thirdly, contrary to Reed's objections to the use of Beckian cognitive therapy with obsessional patients (for example, Beck, 1976), not all of these patients do regard their obsessions and compulsions as absurd (see Sections 1.2.6.2, 1.2.6.3, and 1.3.7); indeed, Reed himself (1985, p. 5) acknowledges that patients report differing degrees of perceived senselessness with respect to their obsessions and compulsions.

6.8 Further comments on Reed's account, and the supporting evidence cited by Reed

6.8.1 The nature of Reed's causal claim

It was pointed out earlier that Reed stresses two points in presenting his thesis – firstly, that the thinking style detailed in his hypothesis is the *primary dysfunction* in obsessional disorders – that is, the cause of the distress experienced by obsessional patients – and secondly, that this thinking style is *general* to the sufferer's functioning. Note that although the first of these statements makes a causal claim, the second does not. The first claim is, furthermore, logically independent of the second. There is no contradiction in the suggestion that a patient's thinking style has caused his distress in some particular area of his functioning, while also supposing that style to be *specific* to that area of the patient's functioning. (Such an account would, of course, beg the question as to why the patient's thinking style is different in that one area, hence the objections to Reed's account considered in Section 6.6.2.)

6.8.2   An explanation of the hypothesised thinking style of obsessionals?

Does Reed also have an explanation for why obsessionals exhibit the thinking style he attributes to them? In an early paper, he introduces this issue but leaves it open: "Given that obsessional thinking does, in fact, reflect a failure in the spontaneous structuring of experience, this failure itself has still to be explained. It is possible to formulate explanatory hypotheses in terms of both psychoanalysis and learning theory. On the other hand, the present hypothesis [i.e., his account] has the merit of encouraging the search for explanations from other viewpoints" (Reed, 1968, p. 291). (These possible behavioural and psychoanalytic accounts Reed mentions would, of course, have to be quite unlike existing behavioural and psychoanalytic accounts, in that they have to explain, consistent with Reed's account, the distress of obsessionals as resulting from their cognitive style.)

None of these possible explanations of the hypothesised cognitive style of obsessionals has been followed up in Reed's subsequent work, and his last full discussion (1985) of both psychoanalytic and behavioural theories contains no suggestion that these approaches might be able to provide such an explanation. This is, of course, a perfectly legitimate position for Reed – having suggested that the distress of obsessionals is an effect of their hypothesised cognitive style, he is not required also to provide an explanation for this cognitive style.

6.8.3   Reed's laboratory tasks

As discussed earlier, Reed attempts to support his account with a number of studies that use laboratory tasks (1969a, 1969b, 1977b), and this work has been followed up by a number of other authors (for example, Volans, 1976; Persons and Foa, 1984; Frost et al., 1988, who used the same task as Persons and Foa; Jakes, 1992, Chapters 5 and 6). These investigations attempt to demonstrate that the thinking style Reed hypothesises to be basic to obsessional disorders can be observed in the performance of obsessional patients (and nonclinical compulsives) on various neutral tasks involving such matters as block sorting, verbal tests and arithmetical problems (*neutral* here means unrelated to the contents of the patient's obsessional difficulties). What would be the significance of obsessionals' performing on these tasks in the manner Reed predicts, and could we infer from such a performance that the thinking style in question *causes* the distress of obsessional patients, as Reed's hypothesis suggests?

The intended argument leading from these tasks to this causal claim can be illustrated by the following example. That an obsessional patient washes her hands, paying close attention to the details of her performance, clearly does not, in itself, confirm Reed's account – this style of performance might be the result, as various types of theorists would indeed argue, of the patient's fearing contact with dirt or germs. A neutral task such as block sorting, the argument continues, does not contain this ambiguity. If the same style of performance can be shown there as is observed on handwashing tasks and the like, then it becomes unparsimonious to explain that style of performance in the case of handwashing in terms specific to that task – such as the patient's having an abnormal fear of contamination. The argument suggests that it is most parsimonious to take this style as the primary dysfunction, consistent with Reed's account, with the observed discomfort as regards handwashing being treated as the effect of the style. (The "trivial and prosaic" contents of some obsessional difficulties, discussed in Section 6.1.1, were supposed by Reed to argue the same point.) This argument, then, attempts to establish one of the claims Reed stresses in presenting his account (that the patient's cognitive style causes her distress) on the basis of the other of these claims (that the patient's cognitive style as observed in her problem areas may also be observed in her behaviour elsewhere).

For the purposes of the present discussion, the premise of this argument – that the cognitive style of obsessional patients is general to their functioning and has been demonstrated to be so by laboratory studies such as Reed's – is taken as given. There are, however, some grounds for doubting this premise. The studies by Reed, Volans, Persons and Foa, and Frost et al. (referred to at the beginning of Section 6.8.3) did indeed all provide some support for Reed's account. However, Jakes (1992, Chapters 5 and 6) tested OCD patients with the three tasks reported by Reed (1969a); Persons and Foa (1984) and Frost et al. (1988); and Volans (1976). Very little support for Reed's account was provided by the performance of OCD patients on any of these tasks in Jakes's investigation. The laboratory evidence is thus equivocal as regards Reed's account.

Even leaving to one side these doubts concerning Reed's premise, one can still fault his argument in at least three separate ways.

OBJECTION (a): PATIENT'S CONCERN ABOUT BEING BLAMED. If the patient's difficulties are hypothesised to stem from some very general concern, such as a fear of being blamed or criticised for making mistakes, then the experimental task may be as relevant to this concern as the everyday tasks and situations that cause the patient's difficulties. According to this objection, that is, the patient may be concerned about being blamed or criticised for making mistakes on the laboratory task, too. This concern, the objection would continue, will produce the observed cognitive style on such tasks, just as it also produces it in the patient's problem areas.

OBJECTION (b): GENERALISATION OF STYLE. A fear, for example of dirt or germs, may have often required the patient, over a long period of time, to make hair-splitting decisions as to whether or not things have been adequately cleaned. This style of dealing with possible sources of contamination, this objection continues, could have generalised from those tasks and situations in which dirt or germs are thought by the patient to be involved, to other tasks and situations (including the laboratory task) where even the patient would agree that dirt and germs are not involved. That is, this style may have become a habit for the patient, no longer tied to serving the ends it was initially introduced to serve. (It is worth noting that it is not the generalising of this style from one area of the patient's life to another per se that is crucial to this objection. It seems that Reed's account could allow for some such generalisation, and indeed, Reed's suggested therapeutic interventions evidently require such generalisations to be possible, albeit in reverse – a reduction in the patient's hypothesised cognitive style is supposed to arise first in the suggested therapeutic exercises and then to spread elsewhere in the patient's functioning. What is crucial to the present objection is that the cognitive style is hypothesised to have arisen in the first place only as a *secondary* phenomenon, as a result of the patient's hypothesised fear of contamination.)

OBJECTION (c): THE PRESENCE OF A PERVASIVE MECHANISM. Patients may exhibit a particular thinking style both in laboratory tasks and in problem areas such as handwashing, as a result of a highly pervasive mechanism such as would be postulated by, for example, some psychodynamic formulations of obsessional difficulties. Thus, such a formulation might suggest that the patient's fear of being unable to control her own anger leads her to displace that anger onto various situations and tasks and then to impose a rigid, detailed order upon – to overstructure, in Reed's terms – these situations and tasks in an attempt to impose symbolic control over her anger. (Also see Sections 5.3 and 5.4.) By assuming that these putative displacement mechanisms are affecting a wide enough range of the patient's thinking and behaviour, one can make sense of the fact that the cognitive style featured in Reed's hypothesis is observed both in the patient's handwashing and in her performance on Reed's laboratory tasks (as well as, of course, in a wide variety of the patient's other behaviour). This third objection implies, along with objection (a), that the patient will not find the laboratory tasks a neutral activity at all, contrary to Reed's assumption.

To demonstrate, then, that an obsessional patient has a distinctive cognitive style that can be observed both within her problem areas and on laboratory tasks, does not show that this style has a causal role in producing the patient's distress. What this observation *would* demonstrate is only that the patient is distinguishable from controls across a sufficiently wide range of her thinking and behaviour for this to be evident in the laboratory tasks. And in the case of some obsessional patients, this demonstration would be neither trivial nor, indeed, easy to make sense of – this would be so particularly for those patients who report only a single obsession and whose difficulties seem relatively isolated within what is evidently an otherwise reasonably normal life (see Section 6.6.2), and those patients whose major difficulties appear not to involve the thinking style hypothesised by Reed at all (see Section 6.6.1). There are other obsessional patients, however, whose difficulties both involve paying close attention to detail and also appear to pervade many things, or even everything, they do. It would be unsurprising to find that the cognitive style of such patients is distinguishable from that of controls on laboratory tasks. Patients with obsessional personality disorders would all have to be of this last kind – a point especially worth noting, as these are the patients with whom Reed conducted his laboratory work.

The foregoing objections (a–c) against attempts to discover the primary dysfunction of obsessionals by means of laboratory tasks can be summarized as follows. (These arguments may also be of relevance to the use of laboratory tasks with other psychiatric groups.) Suppose there are two features – X and Y – that have been observed together, or that have at least been claimed to occur together, in a given psychiatric symptom or given trait of a personality disorder. In the case of obsessionals and Reed's theory, let X be the thinking style described by that theory, and let Y be the patient's emotional distress, be it anxiety, depression, anger or whatever. The use of laboratory tasks is intended to show that X is observable in the absence of Y, rendering, Reed would suggest, the explanation of Y as being caused by X when they are observed together the most parsimonious account of the presence of Y. The foregoing objections (a–c) to this suggestion of Reed's can be summarized, as follows: objection (a) – the claims that Y may be caused by the performance of these laboratory tasks, which in turn causes X to appear on those tasks; objection (b) – the claim that Y does not have to be caused by these laboratory tasks to be the cause of X's appearance on those tasks; and objection (c) – that X and Y may be parallel co-effects of some third variable. (In the example presented, this third variable was the patient's putative fear of, and desire to control, her own anger, this variable being, according to objection [c], what produces, via displacement mechanisms, both the patient's distress as regards cleaning tasks and the like, and her style of dealing with such tasks.)

What, then, if it could be shown that *ex-patients* continue to exhibit the cognitive style postulated by Reed (still assuming for the sake of the present argument that obsessional patients also exhibit this style)? Would this observation confirm Reed's thesis, and would it answer the three objections considered in the foregoing? It would seem not. The observation would certainly be consistent with Reed's position – as noted earlier, he suggests that the cognitive style of obsessionals is a permanent feature of their functioning and that obsessional disorders result from the exacerbation of this feature (although note that Reed's position would thus be inconsistent with patients' and ex-patients' exhibiting *exactly the same* degree of the cognitive style featured in his hypothesis).

Two of the objections considered would, furthermore, have some difficulty in explaining this hypothetical observation with ex-patients. Thus, objection (c) would at least have to explain why its postulated third variable continues to produce in ex-patients the same cognitive style that was exhibited while they were patients, but does not continue to cause the distress they formerly suffered (this distress supposedly being, on this objection, a co-effect of this same variable). Objection (a) would have still more difficulty in explaining this observation. Why should ex-patients continue to be anxious about being criticised for their performance on laboratory tasks – the explanation objection (a) provides of the ex-patient's performance on such tasks – if ex-patients are no longer being troubled by anxieties about being criticised by others in their everyday lives?

But objection (b) would require only minor alterations to accommodate the same observation. Thus, this objection could explain this cognitive style in ex-patients as having generalised from the obsessional difficulties they *once had,* just as, in the case of people currently suffering from obsessional problems, objection (b) explained this style as having generalised from the patient's present difficulties.

The results from laboratory tasks such as Reed's, then, cannot provide strong confirmation of his account. Whether these tasks are conducted with obsessional patients or ex-patients – although particularly in the former case – explanations other than Reed's are available to explain why the thinking style he postulates is observed on such tasks. These tasks thus have a greater potential to disconfirm Reed's thesis than they have to support it. Strong evidence against his account would be provided by a failure to observe the thinking style he hypothesises in the performance of either obsessional patients or ex-patients.

Continuing to assume for the sake of argument, then, that the cognitive style featured in Reed's account is exhibited by obsessional patients, what *would* be reasonable evidence in support of the claim that this style is causing the distress of these patients as regards checking and cleaning tasks and the like?

One important implication of this claim is that changing the thinking style of these patients so that it would be more like that of normal subjects would in turn lead to a reduction in the distress experienced. Investigating whether or not this implication is true would therefore be a crucial test of Reed's thesis and a test that, furthermore, could potentially support Reed's account while disconfirming all three of the objections considered here. Thus, in their various ways, these objections suggest that the thinking style Reed hypothesises obsessional patients to have is either an effect of their distress or its co-effect. All of these objections therefore claim, with Reed, that the thinking style and distress of these patients are associated with one another, while denying, against Reed, that this associa-tion consists of the thinking style's producing the distress. This is, then, why run-ning obsessional patients through laboratory tasks such as Reed's fails to answer any of these objections: this can at most establish only what these objections themselves assert – that the distress of these patients is *associated* with the think-ing style featured in Reed's account. But none of these objections can readily make sense, as Reed's account can, of *manipulations* of this thinking style lead-ing to changes in the level of distress experienced by obsessional patients. If this thinking style is an effect of the patient's distress, or its co-effect, changes in that thinking style should have no effects on the patient's distress (or indeed be impossible without such effects' first being brought about). Another test of Reed's approach would be to attempt a reduction in the obsessional thinking style of ex-patients (assuming here that there are ex-patients who continue to exhibit this style). The crucial observation would be whether the reduction or elimination of this continuing tendency to exhibit this style helps to prevent the subsequent reappearance of obsessional difficulties.

Studies such as those suggested require some means by which to change the hypothesised thinking style of obsessional patients and ex-patients. The therapeutic interventions Reed derives from his hypothesis are one way in which this could be attempted. Given the theoretical importance of such attempts, therefore, the absence of treatment outcome data for these interventions in Reed's (1985) discussion (as noted in Section 6.1.2) is especially regrettable.

Even studies such as those just suggested could not provide very strong evidence that the thinking style of obsessional patients causes their distress. The finding that changing the thinking style of patients reduces their distress would only show that this style *helps maintain* this distress; the finding that changing the thinking style of ex-patients reduces their rate of relapse would only show that this style helps produce the *reappearance* of distress. But either of these findings would make it more plausible to claim that this thinking style causes the distress of obsessional patients and would, in any event, be of clinical value.

One can conclude, then, that the results from laboratory tasks such as Reed's could in themselves provide only strong evidence *against* his theory. If one intended instead to provide strong evidence *in favour* of this theory, the major justification for running such tasks would be that they might provide evidence for the presence of the thinking style Reed postulates, which could then be manipulated in studies such as those suggested.

6.8.4 Evidence for Reed's account based on clinical observations

The foregoing arguments certainly do not mean that there could be no grounds for believing Reed's thesis in the absence of any evidence concerning the outcome of attempts to change the thinking style outlined in that thesis. Reed himself attempts to provide such grounds with his observations that compulsive behaviour increases the discomfort of obsessional patients and that the nature of this discomfort – depression, anger and the like – is such that the discomfort may be very plausibly attributed to the frustration of carrying out these behaviours. Although these observations of Reed's may be disputed (see Sections 6.10 and 6.11), they certainly would, if sound, provide evidence in favour of Reed's analysis.

6.9 Reed's account and the definition of the obsessional personality and personality disorder

As noted in Section 1.2.2, Reed argues that there are clear diagnostic criteria for OCD. As regards the obsessional personality and personality disorder, however, Reed says that "no clear operational definition of [this] has yet evolved" (1985, p. 44) and attempts no definition himself, presenting instead thirty-three traits, such as punctiliousness, indecisiveness and thoroughness, that are most commonly accepted as being among the constituents of this personality/personality disorder.

Yet there is some tension between Reed's theoretical account, and his claim not to have a definition of the obsessional personality and personality disorder. Reed's review of the thirty-three traits most commonly associated with this disorder is followed by his account of these traits in terms of difficulties in "spontaneously structuring" and of the tendency to "overstructure", this account being presented as a "psychological/*semantic* synthesis" (p. 114, emphasis not in original). But if Reed believes that his account picks out a *semantic* link between all obsessional personality traits, why does he not attempt a definition of the obsessional personality disorder as one in which traits exhibiting the features picked out by this account predominate?

6.10   The experience of compulsion

If Reed believes OCD to be a pathological extension of the traits of the obsessional personality disorder, why does his psychological/semantic synthesis of these traits appear to play no part in his account of the defining criteria of OCD (see Section 1.2.2)? Reed's reply to this would probably refer us to his account of what it is for an experience to have "a subjectively compulsive quality". This quality is, in Reed's view (1985, p. 5), the most fundamental of the three defining criteria of OCD he puts forward, and his analysis of it turns out to be closely related to his psychological/semantic synthesis. Quoting several of his patients' accounts of this experience, he suggests that for the most part these accounts do "not stress the *positive strength* of the thoughts, but the *negative strength* of [the patient's] will-power". The experience is characterised, Reed suggests, "not so much by an awareness of a powerful, compelling force as by a feeling of inadequacy in volitional process. The problem seems to be related not to a pathological intensity of *excitation*, but to a relative failure of *inhibition*" (p. 129, original emphasis).

Reed offers some harsh criticisms of theorists – including both behaviourists and psychoanalysts – whose approaches do emphasise, in Reed's terms here, "the power of the thoughts" experienced by patients. The belief in powerful, compelling forces that direct the action of an individual against his own will makes sense most readily, Reed tells us, in a culture that believes in "malign or punitive spirits" (p. 121). This leads Reed to suggest that "it is only a slight exaggeration to claim that contemporary views of obsessional experience savour of medieval thinking" (p. 122). Reed suggests instead that the experience of compulsion may be seen as an imbalance or malfunction in negative feedback, that is, as the poor "spontaneous structuring of experience" detailed in his hypothesis.

Reed's criticisms of accounts that suggest there to be "powerful forces" compelling obsessional patients are certainly unfair. All that this suggestion amounts to is the claim that the sufferer experiences extreme emotion and/or feels highly motivated to act in a certain way. No belief in malign spirits is implied.

There are, in any case, difficulties for Reed's account of the experience of compulsion. If this experience amounts to a "failure of inhibition" in Reed's sense – an imbalance in negative feedback – then, for a thought or action to be attended by this experience, this thought or action would have to occur, or to be performed, *repetitively* – it is this repetitiveness that would be argued by Reed to reflect the patient's failure to inhibit the thought or action. Yet there is no necessity for compulsive thoughts or actions to be repetitive – as noted earlier (see Section 4.4), for example, Rachman and Hodgson (1980) report that compulsive cleaning is often performed without any repetitiveness or doubting.

Commenting on Rachman and Hodgson's (1980) observation that some obsessional patients have no difficulty in deciding when to stop their compulsive behaviour, Reed suggests that the problem of these patients remains one of deciding to act upon their decisions – that is, these patients can decide when they should stop, but they fail to do so (Reed, 1976). But this argument surely misses the point – these patients are reported by Rachman and Hodgson usually to carry out short rituals, so they evidently *can* act on their decisions to stop.

It also seems that Reed's account of obsessional disorders contradicts his analysis of the "experience of compulsion" by virtue of an implication of his account that Reed himself does not acknowledge. This implication is that compulsive behaviours need not always be repetitive. (His account appears similarly to imply that all such behaviours need not always increase discomfort.) Reed's account *does* suggest that compulsions tend to be both discomfort-increasing and prolonged as patients struggle to "structure" any task to their own satisfaction. But Reed's account surely allows that once patients have attained – by "overstructuring" the task – what they regard as a proper or satisfactory way of carrying out the task, subsequent performances of that task need not involve prolonged, discomfort-increasing behaviour. Thus, Reed suggests that thoroughness in the carrying out of some behaviour is one way in which a task may be overstructured (1985, p. 55) – and the thorough performance of some behaviour need not involve that behaviour's being prolonged and accompanied by doubts. (Such thoroughness is similarly consistent with that behaviour's reducing the discomfort of the person who carries it out.) For example, someone may be said to be thorough in keeping a table clean merely because the person removes any slight blemish or speck of dirt as soon as it appears on the table – no repetitiveness or doubting in the performance of this removal is implied.

When one turns to the obsessional personality and personality disorder, still further tensions arise between Reed's account of obsessional disorders and his analysis of the experience of compulsion. Reed argues the traits of this personality and personality disorder not to involve the experience of compulsion at all – it is the absence of this experience, in Reed's view, that helps to distinguish these traits from obsessional symptoms. Yet according to Reed, these traits involve – albeit to a lesser degree than obsessional symptoms – the poor spontaneous structuring of experience (the malfunction in negative feedback) that is central to Reed's analysis of the experience of compulsion.

6.11   The role of anxiety

Reed draws attention to an important point when he stresses that anxiety is not the only mood disturbance observed in obsessional disorders; other workers writing from various perspectives make the same point, for example Beech and Liddell (1974), Beech and Perigault (1974), Rachman and Hodgson (1980), and Claridge (1985). Although all of these authors argue this point on the basis of *phenomenological* evidence, as Reed does, other kinds of data have also been used to defend the related suggestion that OCD should not be classified as an anxiety disorder. Fineberg (1990), for example, points out, in defence of this claim, that OCD differs from anxiety disorders in several (nonphenomenological) ways (see Section 3.6.2).

Reed nonetheless appears to understate the role played by anxiety in obsessional disorders; in particular, his assertion (see Section 6.1.1) that the anxiety of obsessional patients concerns only such questions as, "Will I ever be well?", not questions such as, "Am I dangerously contaminated?" is surely implausible.

6.12   The obsessional personality/personality disorder, OCD and nonobsessional symptoms

As pointed out earlier, Reed's account requires OCD to arise only in the context of an obsessional personality or personality disorder. This does not square with current findings – for example, Black (1974) and Pollack (1979, 1987). (This raises the interesting and little-researched question of how, if at all, the obsessional symptoms of patients who do have obsessional personalities differ from those of patients with other personality types.)

Reed is explicit that his account of obsessional disorders treats the mood disturbance observed in them as secondary and thus sharply distinguishes them from depressive and anxiety disorders. How does Reed make sense, then, of the link between obsessional and depressive disorders, given Lewis's (1936) claim that this link cannot to be explained in terms only of the depressing nature of obsessional disorders? Support for Lewis's position is provided by Gittleson's (1966) observation that some patients experience an emergence of, or increase in, obsessions only after they have become depressed. Reed (1985, p. 143) suggests that this observation may reflect a "spreading effect"; with a general lowering of resistance in depression, he argues, a wider range of obsessions may intrude. But why should one suppose that "low resistance" leads to the intrusion of obsessions? (This appears to be an especially surprising claim for Reed to make, given his diagnostic criterion that all obsessions must be resisted.)

Reed's account also has difficulty in explaining the co-morbidity of OCD with anxiety disorders such as simple phobias, social phobias, agoraphobias, panic disorder and separation anxiety (Rasmussen and Tsuang, 1986). This co-morbidity suggests there to be some overlap in the mechanisms that produce these various disorders, yet Reed's account explicitly leaves no room for such an overlap.

6.13   External structuring

Reed (1968) reports that the compulsive behaviour of some obsessionals is reduced by the presence, reassurance and/or intervention of a trusted person. This enables the patient, Reed points out (1968, 1985), to delegate decisions and responsibilities. But what Reed does not explain is why this delegation of decisions and responsibility should be of help. The problems that Reed suggests are encountered by obsession-als in determining the answers to questions such as, "Did I do it properly?" should be no greater than those encountered in answering questions such as, "Has this other person done it properly?" (Jakes, 1987).

Indeed, rather than supporting Reed's account, the observation that obsession-als benefit from the delegation of decisions and responsibilities would suggest that their problems relate instead to doubts specifically about themselves and their own action. (It could similarly be argued that such doubts are also present in the contents of some obsessional symptoms – for example, those in which the patient checks or ruminates as to whether or not he has performed some violent act [Jakes, 1987]).

This phenomenon of being helped by the presence, reassurance and/or inter-vention of a trusted person is exhibited by only *some* obsessionals (Stern and Cobb, 1978; also see Jakes, 1992, Chapter 2). It would be of interest to know if this fea-ture bears any relationship to Lewis's (1936) distinction, discussed earlier, between obstinate and irritable obsessional personalities on the one hand, and vacillating and submissive obsessional personalties on the other. Is it only the latter who tend to seek the reassurance and help of others? And does the obstinacy of the former group tend to produce precisely the opposite profile, of having to do things for one-self and being unable to trust others to do them properly? Evidence possibly of rel-evance to these questions is provided by Rachman and Hodgson (1980, p. 54), who report checkers to be both more likely than cleaners to seek reassurance and also more likely than cleaners to have a vacillating and uncertain personality profile.

6.14   Reed's account of Janet

Reed argues that his formulation of obsessional disorders has much in common with Janet's account of psychasthenia. Some comments on this are offered else-where (Section 4.5), but it is worth noting here that among other difficulties fac-ing this interpretation is the fact that Janet includes various disorders in addition to OCD under the common rubric of psychasthenia – including what would nowadays be diagnosed as agoraphobia, social phobia and panic disorder (see Section 4.2) – and endeavours to explain all of them, along with OCD, in terms of a lowering of the sufferer's psychological tension (see Section 4.4). This is in clear contrast, then, to Reed's own account, which is intended to apply specifically to obsessional disorders and is unable to explain, as noted in Section 6.12, the co-morbidity of OCD with these other disorders.

6.15 Summary

Reed originally argued that obsessional disorders all stem from difficulties in the spontaneous structuring of experience, which leads to compensatory over-structuring. Reed himself later pointed out that this hypothesis, as it stood, made poor sense of some cases – especially, it seemed, those involving checking and rumination. He introduced the redintegration supplement in an attempt to remedy this, but the supplement turns out to be implausible. Reed's hypothesis has also been argued to make poor sense of obsessional difficulties in which doubts, indecision and ritualising do not play a major role or do not appear at all. Certain aspects of some obsessional difficulties that *do* involve these features, furthermore, are not explained by this account – particularly, certain themes' being observed in many cases, and these difficulties' sometimes involving just a few areas of the patient's life.

It has been argued that Reed's hypothesis also fails to explain the *motivation* of obsessionals in carrying out their compulsive behaviour. A revised version of Reed's thesis was suggested that can explain why at least some obsessionals are highly motivated to behave as they do, but this thesis fails to account for various observations, especially – once again – those that tend to be associated with checking difficulties. It was argued that a *partial* explanation of such difficulties from this perspective may be possible, however. This Revised Thesis was also argued to be poor at distinguishing obsessionals from other psychiatric groups, including phobic and deluded subjects.

The evidence based on laboratory tasks that Reed has presented in favour of his thesis, it has been argued, can provide only weak support, and the clinical observations Reed cites to this same end are at best controversial. It has also been suggested that the existing evidence from such tasks is equivocal as regards Reed's account. Objections have also been brought against Reed's comments regarding the use of assertiveness training and behavioural and cognitive therapy with obsessionals.

It has been argued that Reed's account misrepresents the role of anxiety in obsessional disorders and carries implausible implications as to the relationship both between OCD and the obsessional personality/personality disorder and between OCD, on the one hand, and anxiety and depressive disorders on the other.

A number of comments have been offered on Reed's discussion of external structuring, his interpretation of Janet, his account of the experience of compulsion and his comments on the definition of OCD and of the obsessional personality and personality disorder.

What of Reed's account may be salvaged from the foregoing discussion? The account appears to be most plausible when regarded as a *partial* explanation of *some* obsessional difficulties, in particular those where one observes the patient's having, in Reed's terms, problems structuring some task and tending to perform it in an overstructured manner. Among the best examples of cases of this kind appear to be at least some instances involving contamination fears and cleaning behaviour (see the example of handwashing discussed in Section 6.1.1).

The Revised Thesis seems most likely to provide a full explanation in the case of those obsessional difficulties in which some unlikely outcome is feared by the patient, but in which neither constant doubts about, nor endless repetitions of, compulsive behaviours are observed. Many cases involving cleaning difficulties correspond to this profile.

Both Reed's account and the Revised Thesis, therefore, seem to be most plausible in the case of many instances of cleaning difficulties. It needs to be stressed, however, that the greater plausibility of these approaches as regards cleaning problems really amounts to no more than the absence of the objections that arise regarding the application of Reed's account and the Revised Thesis to other kinds of difficulties, such as checking behaviours and discrete obsessional thoughts, images and impulses. There are, that is, no positive grounds for accepting either of these approaches even in the case of cleaning problems, and it remains entirely possible, therefore, that the cognitive factors reviewed in this chapter will turn out to be entirely secondary phenomena in obsessional disorders, playing only a minor, or even no, role – if they appear at all – in producing the pathological thinking and behaviour that is observed.

7 Biological approaches to OCD

7.1 Introduction

An increase of interest has recently been shown in biological approaches to OCD, and there are available a number of reviews/discussions of the findings from genetic, neuroanatomical, neurophysiological, neuropsychological and biochemical studies of OCD, as well as from studies of what have been presented as animal models of the disorder (for example, Turner, Beidel and Nathan, 1985; Rapoport and Wise, 1988; Insel, 1988; Pitman, 1989). This chapter will attempt to offer neither detailed comments on the quality of these biological findings, nor a comprehensive review of them. Instead, some of what have been claimed to be the most important of these findings will be briefly outlined, along with some of the suggestions biological theorists have offered regarding the psychological processes at work in OCD. Discussion will then focus on how powerful an argument in favour of a biological account of OCD these findings, if sound, could sustain.

Given the use of supposed animal models of OCD in some biological research, a few remarks concerning such models are in order here. (Animal models of OCD are also offered in other types of research – for example, de Silva, 1988, pp. 206–7). Reed (1985, p. 11) objects to the use of animal models in the study of OCD on the basis of his belief that the defining criteria for the disorder are *phenomenological* – for a thought or action to be symptomatic of the disorder, according to Reed, it must be experienced as senseless and be resisted, and it is unclear, in the case of any animal behaviour, on what grounds it could be argued that such behaviour has been experienced in this way (although see de Silva, 1988, p. 207). Against Reed's position, however, it is not necessary for all OCD symptoms to be experienced as senseless and to be resisted (see Chapter 1), and even if this were the case, surely there still remains an open question of whether or not an animal's behaviour is sufficiently like that of an OCD patient in other respects (for example, the context in which it is provoked, what is done in carrying out the behaviour) for it to be useful as at least a partial model of that behaviour.

Note that some work that might be classified as biological – in particular, that of Gray (see Chapter 3) – has already been discussed.

7.2 The work of Rapoport and Wise, and Insel

Rapoport and Wise (1988, p. 382) have put forward a neural model of OCD, an adapted version of which has been presented by Insel (1988). This model places particular emphasis on the role of a "four–neuron loop" in OCD (Rapoport and Wise, 1988, p. 381), consisting of projections (1) from the cortex to the striatum, (2) from the striatum to the globus pallidus, (3) from the globus pallidus to the thalamus and (4) from the thalamus back to the cortex.

This model is illustrated in Figure 7.1, which is taken from Insel (1988, p. 368); Insel's explanatory remarks are quoted in full.

Rapoport and Wise (1988) further note that a high concentration of serotonin and serotonin receptors have been found in the basal ganglia, and they suggest that "the striatal serotonin system potentiates, by excitatory modulation, [the] inputs to the striatum" that feature in their model (p. 381). This concentration of serotonin receptors in the basal ganglia means that evidence suggesting a possible role for serotonergic mechanisms in OCD, on the one hand, and evidence indicating the possible involvement of the basal ganglia in the disorder, on the other, may be to some extent mutually supportive.

Rapoport and Wise (1988) and Insel (1988) argue that a number of findings are consistent with the hypothesis that both this four-neuron loop and the striatal serotonin system have a central role in OCD. Thus, in support of the involvement of this four-neuron loop, Insel (1988, p. 368) cites improvements in OCD that have been reported following surgical interruption of frontal-striatal pathways; the atrophy of the caudate nucleus in OCD patients (Luxenberg et al., 1986 –

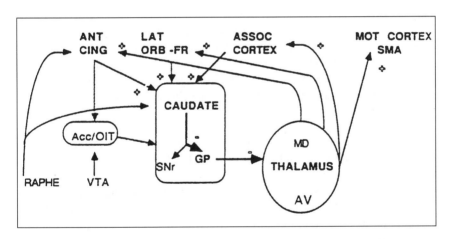

Figure 7.1 Model of circuits linking cortex and basal ganglia. This cartoon of the afferents to and efferents from basal ganglia depicts some of the circuits that have been implicated in displacement behavior or stereotypy in mammals. The central point is that globus pallidus (GP) output is inhibitory for anterior ventral (AV) and mediodorsal (MD) thalmus. In obsessive-compulsive disorder, decreased GP output could result in increased activity of the positive feedback circuits from these thalmic nuclei to motor (MOT) cortex (possibly resulting in excessive motor behavior) and lateral-orbital-frontal (LAT-ORB-FR) cortex (possibly resulting in increased worry, anxiety, obsessions). Note that serotonergic input to this system might provide a locus for pharmacologic intervention and that surgically interrupting cingulate (ANT CING) and frontal pathways to the striatum has been observed to decrease obsessional symptoms. SMA = supplementary motor area; Acc/OIT = nucleus accumbens, olfactory tubercle; SNr = substantia nigra; VTA = ventral tegmental area. (Insel, 1988, p. 368)

although only a normal control group was included in this study); and the increase in metabolic rate in both the frontal cortex and the basal ganglia in OCD patients, as compared with both unipolar depressed patients and normal controls (Baxter et al., 1987). (A number of further neuro-imaging studies comparing OCD patients with normal controls are cited by Hymas et al., 1991, p. 2224, Table 7.)

Rapoport (1989, p. 66) argues that basal ganglia involvement in OCD is further indicated by the disorder's occurring in association with several neurological disorders, all of which are known to involve damage to this area – for example, Sydenham's chorea, epilepsy, postencephalitic Parkinson's disease, and toxic lesions of the basal ganglia. Rapoport (1989) also suggests that 20% of her sample of OCD patients showed "chorea-like twitches" and that "standard tests designed to identify specific neurological function indicate that [these] patients have functional deficits in the frontal lobes or the basal ganglia or both" (p. 66).

As regards the suggested role of serotonin in OCD, Rapoport (1989, p. 64) argues that this is confirmed by the efficacy of clomipramine, fluvoxamine and fluoxetine (all of which block the reuptake of serotonin) in ameliorating OCD. Zohar et al. (1988) add that another serotonin reuptake blocker, zimelidine, has also been reported to be an effective treatment for OCD. Zohar et al. (1987) note that OCD is exacerbated by the administration of metachlorophenylpiperazine (mCPP), a selective serotonin agonist, and Zohar et al. (1988) have shown that this effect is decreased by clomipramine treatment. Zohar et al. (1988) argue, on the basis of these observations, that OCD may be associated with increased serotonergic activity and that chronic treatment with serotonergic reuptake blockers may induce *down-regulation* of serotonergic responsiveness (that is, induce serotonergic subsensitivity). Consistent with this position, Zohar et al. (1988) note that an exacerbation of OCD symptoms may be reported during the first few days of clomipramine treatment. Insel et al. (1983) further report an elevation in the levels of the serotonin metabolite 5-HIAA in the cerebrospinal fluid of OCD patients.

7.3   Further evidence of relevance to the work of Rapoport and Wise and to the work of Insel

Hymas et al. (1991) report neurological, motor and neuropsychological examinations of seventeen OCD patients exhibiting what these authors term *obsessional slowness* (a phenomenon originally described by Rachman [1974] as "Primary Obsessional Slowness", although Hymas et al. [p. 2205] note what they take to be some inconsistencies in Rachman's description of obsessional slowness). Hymas et al. introduce their study by describing an OCD patient whose slowness, they claim, resulted from such difficulties as "initiating simple movements" and "shifting between...different patterns of movement", making this patient's deficits "reminiscent of...for example, frontal lobe disorders, or Parkinson's disease"(p. 2205). Consistent with this, Hymas et al. (p. 2225) report their sample of OCD patients to exhibit "motor and cognitive impairments consistent with the hypothesis that functions served by frontal and basal ganglia mechanisms might be impaired" (although only a normal control group was included in Hymas et al.'s study, and motor and other neurological ratings were not conducted blind). Hymas et al. point out that these findings are consistent with those reported in (1) various single-case reports involving patients in whom disturbance of the frontal cortex and basal ganglia have been accompanied by "obsessive-compulsive phenomena" (p. 2224; see p. 2223, Table 6, for these case reports) and (2) "several systematic studies" of OCD patients not selected for neurological abnormality, including the studies by Luxenberg et al. and Baxter et al. previously discussed (see Hymas et al., p. 2224, Table 7). The fact that Hymas et al.'s results are consistent with these studies, which were conducted with OCD patients not selected for "slowness", surely suggests that these authors may be placing too much importance upon the supposed similarities between their "obsessionally slow" patients on the one hand, and patients suffering from disorders known to involve frontal or basal ganglia mechanisms on the other, in making their case for the involvement of these mechanisms in the pathology of these "slow" OCD patients.

7.4   Gilles de la Tourette syndrome and OCD

Cummings and Frankel (1985) also suggest that OCD may involve abnormal neurophysiological activity in "subcortical forebrain structures (particularly the basal ganglia)" (p. 1119), arguing for this on the basis of (1) the evidence for the involvement of abnormal activity in these structures in Gilles de la Tourette syndrome (GTS) and (2) the various links between GTS and OCD. Concerning the neurological basis of GTS, Cummings and Frankel's arguments are in part similar to those of Rapoport and Wise (1988) and Insel (1988) as regards OCD. Thus, they emphasise, in particular, the association between GTS and known basal ganglia disorders, and also what they suggest – in contrast to OCD – to be the indications of abnormal *dopamine* function in GTS (for example, GTS's responding favourably to haloperidol and other dopamine-blocking agents); they point out that dopamine is located primarily in the basal ganglia and limbic regions (Cummings and Frankel, 1985, p. 1118).

Among the links between OCD and GTS that are picked out by Cummings and Frankel are the large number of GTS patients who also report OCD, the increased occurrence of OCD among GTS family members, and the occurrence of both OCD and GTS in association with certain neurological conditions (for example, postencephalitic states). Cummings and Frankel do not discuss the important matter of the prevalence of tics and GTS among OCD patients, and Green and Pitman (1986, p. 150) suggest that "little...attention has been paid to this question", although Green and Pitman also note that there have been occasional reports of the occurrence of tics in OCD patients (Rapoport's report of "twitches" among her OCD patients has already been noted). Green and Pitman further suggest that Janet (1903) reported the illness of "15 of his 325 obsessive-compulsive cases to have begun with tics" (Green and Pitman, 1986, p. 150; however, not all of these 325 cases had OCD – see Chapter 4).

Some care may be required regarding the interpretation of these associations between tics or GTS and OCD. Green and Pitman argue that in patients with both tics and compulsions, "it was sometimes impossible to tell where one ended and the other began" and that, in particular, a "subjective sense of control, a feature which distinguishes classical descriptions of [GTS] and OCD, could not be used to separate tics from compulsions. Several [GTS] patients reported that they experienced themselves as the voluntary agent of their movements and noises" (pp. 157–8). Green and Pitman suggest (p. 152) that a diagnosis of OCD rather than GTS "may reflect the patient's willingness or ability to verbalize semi-rational explanations for irrational behaviour" – that is, the behaviour seen in some tics and the behaviour seen in some compulsions may, on this view, be fundamentally the same, distinguished only by the extent to which the patient has rationalised its performance.

In contrast to this view, Cummings and Frankel (1985) note that "premovement potentials" have been reported to be absent prior to the tics of GTS patients, suggesting that these movements are "not volitionally initiated in cortical regions and must originate in subcortical structures". Perhaps, then, at least two quite different kinds of movement tend to be classified as tics. If this is so, the finding that there are associations between OCD and tics or GTS is ambiguous – in any given case, this might represent the co-occurrence of two quite distinct phenomena, but equally, it might not. (Further comments will be offered presently as regards Cummings and Frankel's account of the distinction between tics and compulsions.)

Cummings and Frankel also point out that there are certain similarities between the presentations of OCD and GTS – for example, both sharing "the same bizarre sexual, aggressive, and visceral-eliminative themes", both being worsened by anxiety and depression, and both being "lifelong, waxing and waning disorders that begin early in life and are ameliorated by age" (p. 1120).

On the basis of all these observations, Cummings and Frankel suggest that biological abnormalities somewhat similar to those they hypothesise in the case of GTS may also help account for the symptoms of OCD. They suggest that this hypothesis is most applicable to OCD that occurs in conjunction with, or in the context of a family history of, GTS but that it might possibly extend to cases of OCD that have neither of these associations with GTS.

Finally, Cummings and Frankel stress the differences between GTS and OCD – in particular, the absence of tics and vocalisations in the symptomatology of OCD, and what Cummings and Frankel present as the contrasting biochemical profiles observed in the two disorders (the predominant role of dopaminergic mechanisms in GTS, and serotonergic mechanisms in OCD). Cummings and Frankel raise the possibility that these differences may themselves be associated, both reflecting "differences in the level of motor-behavioural organisation that is most involved" in the two disorders.

7.5   The work of Pitman

Pitman (1989), in a review of animal models of compulsive behaviour, also suggests that the basal ganglia may be involved in OCD although, contrary to the suggestions considered so far, he argues that it is *an excess of dopaminergic activity* in this area that is the common denominator of the models he considers (p. 189). (When attempting to reconcile this position with what is known about OCD patients, however, Pitman only notes as "paradoxes" such observations as dopamine antagonists' not being effective in treating OCD and the indirect dopamine agonist, amphetamine, having been reported in at least one study to improve the disorder.)

Pitman also suggests that there may be a role for the limbic system in OCD, both Jenike (1984) and Gray (1982) also having argued for the importance of this system in explaining the disorder (also see Chapter 3). In Pitman's view, a reduction of the limbic system's influence over the basal ganglia may help to account for OCD. He postulates (p. 194) that the junction of these two systems (that is, the "limbic striatum" – and, in particular, the nucleus accumbens) may be the site where this influence is ordinarily exercised, and he notes that this area is among those accorded a role in OCD by Insel and by Rapoport and Wise.

7.6   Psychological accounts offered by biological approaches

Within the accounts outlined in this chapter, a number of suggestions are offered about the psychological processes in terms of which OCD may be explained and about the way in which these processes relate to the brain mechanisms detailed in these accounts.

THE DISPLACEMENT/CONFLICT ACCOUNT. Insel (1988) suggests that family conflict concerning power or control is common for OCD patients; he also argues that "aggressive impulses and guilt are certainly associated with most compulsive rituals" (p. 368). He goes on to note, however, that many people suffer conflict of the kind OCD patients report, without developing the disorder themselves (also see Section 5.4.3 and Chapter 8). Insel suggests that a source for individual differences in the response to such conflict may lie "in the neural substrates noted for 'normal' ritualistic behaviours in other mammals", which turn out to be among the structures included in his, and Rapoport and Wise's, model. Insel argues that these ritualistic behaviours in other mammals – the so-called displacement behaviours – are triggered or released in animals by conflict and may be decreased by lesions of the globus pallidus. There may also be, Insel further suggests, a link between such behaviour and serotonergic function. He also notes "a considerable (although not entirely consistent) literature linking serotonin to aggression" (p. 366). Insel discusses "adjunctive behaviour" as having "some of the qualities of displacement" (p. 366) and notes that such behaviour may be reduced by 6-hydroxydopamine lesions of the nucleus accumbens.

THE DOUBTING/SCEPTICAL ACCOUNT.   An alternative account, making reference to the same brain mechanisms, is outlined by Insel in the same paper (1988). He argues that it is "equally plausible [to postulate]...a neural deficit involving the resolution of doubt" in order to explain OCD; a neural circuit that may be relevant to this, he suggests, includes the basal ganglia. (He also notes, following Gray [1982] that the hippocampus may be an alternative or additional structure that is concerned with the resolution of doubt; also see Chapter 3.) Rapoport (1989) and Rapoport and Wise (1988) similarly suggest that the basal ganglia may be involved in the resolution of doubt. Rapoport (1989, p. 66) suggests that the basal ganglia "are known to be 'way stations' between sensory inputs and the resulting motor or cognitive outputs" and that OCD may result from a short circuit of "the loop that normally connects [such] sensory input with behavioural outputs", leading, according to Rapoport, to the compulsive cleaning and checking (and also, seemingly, the doubting) that feature in the symptoms of OCD patients. She suggests that the OCD patient with cleaning or checking difficulties is "in a Berkleyan nightmare" (Rapoport and Wise, 1988, p. 383) – the patient "becomes an ultimate skeptic who cannot credit his sense data" (Rapoport, 1989, p. 69) – and she similarly suggests that ruminating OCD patients are "skeptics who doubt...their own reasoning" (Rapoport and Wise, 1988, p. 383).

These two approaches to OCD – the displacement/conflict account and the doubting/sceptical account – are clearly distinguishable. The doubting/sceptical approach does not predict that any conflict would be apparent in the patient's dealings with other people, except from that which occurs *because* of his symptoms, and it may be that the doubting/sceptical approach less readily explains the *selectivity* (see Sections 2.2, 3.4 and 3.5) of the thinking, fears and behaviour seen in OCD than does the displacement/conflict account. The displacement/conflict account suggests that this selectivity occurs because such thinking, fears and behaviour are the "fixed action patterns" (Insel, 1988, p. 366) for our species in conditions of conflict. On the doubting/sceptical account, however, it seems that many or all of the patient's thoughts and behaviours ought to be subject to obsessional doubts and compulsive performance. Rapoport and Wise (1988) acknowledge this difficulty when they remark that their approach "fails to account for...[the] behavioural specificity [of OCD]", but elsewhere, outlining the same neuropsychological model, Rapoport (1989) argues that the behaviours of OCD patients "seem to resemble...fixed action patterns" (p. 65) and that "ritualistic behaviour...appears to be hard-wired into the brain" (p. 69). These claims appear to be borrowed from the displacement/conflict account, with little or no explanation offered as to how they can be integrated into the doubting/sceptical approach.

Other objections to the doubting/sceptical account may be possible. It was argued in Section 6.3 that accounts of OCD must be able to explain why the proper completion of, for example, checking and cleaning tasks *matters* more to OCD patients than to others. It is insufficient, on this objection, for accounts merely to explain why it might be more difficult for such patients to *establish that* tasks have been so completed, yet this is the only difficulty that Rapoport and Wise's model appears to address. There are, furthermore, many OCD symptoms that do not involve doubts or indecision at all (see Chapter 1), and the doubting/sceptical account seems to be silent as to the explanation of these symptoms.

Turning now to the displacement/conflict account, Insel himself offers the observation against this account that displacement behaviours in animals are "potent social signals" (1988, p. 366), whereas OCD patients are notoriously secretive about their symptoms. This, Insel suggests, may be contrary to his earlier characterisation of displacement behaviour, in which he suggested links between such behaviour and compulsions in humans. As well as emphasising a difference between displacement behaviour and compulsions, this observation of Insel's also calls into question his suggested link between displacement behaviour and serotonergic function, which was based on (1) displacement behaviour's being "woven into the fabric of social status" (p. 366) and (2) measures of serotonergic function having been correlated with social status in several primate species (p. 366).

Insel (1988) suggests that displacement behaviour resembles compulsions both in its *form* (that is, being out of context and excessive [p. 365], and in its *content* (the cleaning, hoarding and checking of OCD patients involving, that is, actions similar to those seen in displacement behaviour [p. 366]; see later, however, for further points on Insel's views regarding the content of OCD symptoms). Yet this suggested similarity of content may be missing in the case of the behaviours that have been eliminated by means of lesions of the globus pallidus and nucleus accumbens in the studies Insel cites. Thus, lesions of the globus pallidus eliminated displacement "vocalisation...and penile erection" in squirrel monkeys (p. 366), and lesions of the nucleus accumbens eliminated adjunctive drinking in rats. (See Pitman, 1983, for a comparison of the effects of globus pallidus lesions with the symptoms of a GTS patient. Perhaps these effects might also be compared, in some respects, with some OCD fears and impulses. Pitman [1989] also attempts to compare adjunctive drinking with the behaviour of some eating-disorder patients.) It seems that Insel's model predicts that lesions of the globus pallidus, and perhaps of the nucleus accumbens too, should produce an *increase* in displacement behaviour and OCD. Thus, he argues that globus pallidus output "is inhibitory for [the] anterior ventral...and mediodorsal...thalamus" and that a decrease in globus pallidus output may therefore result in "excessive motor behaviour...anxiety [and] obsessions" (1988, p. 368, Figure 7; also see Section 7.2).

Perhaps Insel would reply to the foregoing points concerning the content of some of the displacement behaviour he discusses by somewhat altering the position attributed to him earlier, and by instead emphasising a point he also makes, that the particular actions that become displacement behaviour "are typical within a species but vary greatly between species" (1988, p. 365). This would enable him to argue that it is the out-of-context, excessive nature of displacement behaviour (its *form*), not the specific actions that feature in that behaviour (its *content*), that is the most important aspect of the animal models he discusses.

It is of interest to compare this reply with the position argued in Section 3.4 regarding attempts to explain OCD symptoms from an evolutionary perspective (de Silva et al., 1977; Gray, 1982). Although such a perspective, it was suggested, may be able to explain the content of some OCD symptoms, it is less successful at accounting for the excessive and repetitive nature (as well as various other features) of the fears and behaviour of some OCD patients. The position of this evolutionary perspective is, thus, the exact reverse of that suggested for Insel's displacement/conflict account in the reply that has just been outlined.

It is also worth noting that although being repetitive and stereotyped may render displacement behaviours similar in form to *some* compulsions, it also suggests that they are quite unlike *other* compulsions. Cleaning compulsions, in particular, tend to exhibit neither characteristic (Rachman and Hodgson, 1980), as previously discussed (for example, Section 2.5).

These objections do not seem to entirely undermine Insel's displacement/conflict account, and further support for this account may be available from clinical sources. Thus, although the term *displacement behaviour* may be suspect in some circumstances (see Section 4.5.6), the symptoms of some OCD patients, consistent with Insel's emphasis on the importance of conflict over aggression, may arise in response to the difficulties some of these patients have in asserting themselves and also may perhaps be reduced when these patients become more assertive (also see Sections 4.7.3 and 5.3.2, and Chapter 8).

Still further suggestions as to the psychological processes involved in OCD, and the relationship between these processes and the basal ganglia (and the limbic system) are offered by Pitman (1989). Indeed, his discussion advances a variety of accounts of these processes without fully acknowledging the differences between these accounts. Pitman, following Mishkin, Malamut and Bachevalier (1984), proposes the existence of a *habit system*, responsible for the "slow formation of noncognitive stimulus–response (S–R) bonds through reinforcement" (Pitman, 1989, p. 190), and a *memory system*, which "limits the activity of the habit system" and promotes greater "behavioural variability" (p. 193). The basal ganglia, in Pitman's view, mediate the activities of the habit system, and the limbic system mediates those of the memory system. Pitman hypothesises that the influence of the memory system over the habit system is attenuated in OCD. As Pitman remarks, it is of interest to contrast the role this account assigns the limbic/memory system with the role it is assigned by Gray (1982). Whereas, on Gray's account, "hippocampus-generated behavioural inhibition represents a symptom" (Pitman, 1989, p. 193; also see Chapter 3), on Pitman's view "it represents a potential, but failed cure" (1989, p. 193).

Pitman attempts to support his hypothesis (that the influence of the memory system over the habit system is attenuated in OCD) with reference to a number of animal models and other evidence. Thus, he suggests that the hippocampus has been found in animal experiments to attenuate "the stereotypy-inducing effect of reward" and that electrical stimulation of reinforcement mechanisms in rodents produces behaviour characterised by its "stereotyped performance, excessiveness, resistance to extinction, and divorce from consummatory process" (p. 191). Human compulsive behaviour, Pitman suggests, exhibits similar characteristics. Pitman further notes the important role assigned to negative reinforcement by behavioural accounts of OCD and suggests that when the hippocampus and amygdala are removed in primates, it has been shown that learning becomes "everything for which early S–R theorists could have wished" (p. 190). Pitman suggests that this evidence all points toward OCD's reflecting the formation of habits by basal ganglia mechanisms unmodified by the operation of the memory/limbic system.

Pitman's argument here seems illegitimately to equate the "noncognitive stimulus–response bonds" formed in the absence of the hippocampus and amygdala with the stereotyped and excessive behaviours induced by reward in animals (and humans) in which (and in whom) the hippocampus and amygdala are intact. Moreover, it is surely the behaviour of those animals that have been deprived of these limbic structures that Pitman, on his account of the physical basis of OCD, would be most justified in claiming to be a model of the disorder. Yet the removal of these structures produces only behaviour that reflects, according to Pitman, the formation of "noncognitive stimulus–response bonds", the plausibility of which as a model of compulsive behaviour seems questionable; this behaviour lacks, for example, the stereotyped and excessive nature that was noted by Pitman as regards reward-induced behaviours and that was stressed by Insel in his account of OCD, as noted earlier.

Pitman's position is complicated still further by his also suggesting, on the basis of other work with animals, that the basal ganglia may act as a cybernetic "control system" (p. 192). Pitman links this suggestion with his cybernetic model of OCD, which was discussed in Section 4.9. Yet it is surely arguable that this cybernetic account of OCD may be difficult to reconcile with Pitman's suggestion that the disorder reflects the formation of habits unmodified by the memory/limbic system. And it also seems difficult to reconcile either of these two approaches with the displacement/conflict account. (Note, however, that there may be links between Pitman's cybernetic model and the doubting/sceptical account of Insel and of Rapoport and Wise; also see Section 4.9.3.1.) The picture that begins to emerge here, then, does not consist of various observations and suggestions converging to support a unitary model of OCD. This impression is reinforced by Pitman's further suggestions that the "sensory functions of the basal ganglia" produce both the "sensory precursors to tic...noted in 88% of [GTS] patients" (p. 191) and some of the sensory and ideational precursors reported in many instances of compulsive behaviour. Perhaps a unitary psychological model of OCD may, then, have to be abandoned by biological theorists in favour of a number of different accounts, each applying to only some instances of the disorder. Alternatively, perhaps at least some of the observations and suggestions reviewed in this section may have to be rejected as irrelevant to OCD.

To sum up, these various, evidently conflicting, accounts of the psychological processes that are involved in OCD must be regarded at best as provisional formulations of the disorder, with Insel's displacement/conflict account's being that which might be argued to be at present most promising. The suggestions these accounts offer as to the functions performed by various brain structures must also be regarded as provisional.

7.7   A causal role in OCD for the basal ganglia and the other brain structures discussed by biological approaches

What, then, of the involvement in OCD of the basal ganglia and the other brain structures discussed by the foregoing biological accounts, leaving to one side here the neuropsychology of these structures? How confident should one be that abnormalities in these structures (and particularly those discussed by Rapoport and Wise and by Insel) play some role in *causing* at least some cases of OCD?

This question should perhaps be clarified a little (also see Section 3.7.1). To establish that some brain mechanism plays a part in causing OCD, in the sense of *cause* that is intended here, would be to show that (1) there are differences between this mechanism in OCD patients and the mechanism in normal controls and (2) these differences are involved in mediating the symptoms of OCD. (It would evidently *not* be necessary to show that OCD patients differ from *psychiatric* controls in respect to this mechanism; the mechanism might be the cause – or part of the cause – of both OCD and other psychiatric disorders.) Some brain mechanism's playing a part in causing OCD should also be understood to involve either that mechanism's helping to *produce* OCD (that is, its helping to bring about the onset of the disorder) or that mechanism's helping to *maintain* the disorder. To establish (1) and (2) would not, of course, explain how the observed difference between the relevant brain mechanism in OCD patients and in normal controls came about, and some further remarks on this point are required.

The term *abnormality* will be used in what follows (and has been used at the beginning of this section) to refer to supposed differences between the brains of OCD patients and those of normal controls; the use of this term is intended to carry no implications regarding the question of the origin(s) of these supposed differences.

Is it the case, then, that abnormalities in brain structures such as the basal ganglia play a role in causing OCD? Do such abnormalities play some role in producing, and in maintaining, the disorder? As emphasised, the present chapter has offered neither detailed nor comprehensive scrutiny of the biological findings discussed in connection with OCD. Therefore, no firm answers can be provided here regarding the foregoing questions. The less ambitious aim here is rather to assess whether or not the observations offered by the foregoing biological theories would, if sound, support suggestions that such abnormalities do play this role.

Observations such as the atrophy of the caudate nucleus and increased metabolic rates in the basal ganglia (and frontal cortex) of OCD patients, and findings such as those reported by Hymas et al., could certainly not, in themselves, establish these differences between OCD patients and others to be the whole cause, or part of the cause, of the disorder. These differences between OCD patients and others are, in themselves, no more likely to be involved in causing OCD than they are to be its effects or to be co-effects with OCD (the latter indicating that both the disorder and these supposed differences between OCD patients and others are produced by some further variable[s]).

How might one distinguish between these possibilities? Some progress could be made here by attempting to *manipulate* the suggested abnormalities in OCD patients regarding the brain mechanisms in question, to see if this had any impact on the reported symptoms. If these supposed abnormalities were an effect of, or a co-effect with, OCD, then a reduction of (or compensation for) these abnormalities should make no difference to the disorder (or should even be impossible without an improvement in the disorder having been brought about first). An intervention's leading to a reduction of, or compensation for, these abnormalities would of course have to be identified on grounds other than whether or not that intervention produced an improvement in OCD symptoms, otherwise the statement that this reduction or compensation had had this effect would be tautological. It appears best for these purposes to identify an intervention's effects in physical terms – its observed effects on the brain mechanisms in question. For example, if some brain mechanism X were found in OCD patients to have a greater than normal excitatory input into some second brain mechanism Y, one would wish to know if an intervention that led to a reduction in the severity of the OCD of these patients reduced the excitatory output of X or, if not, reversed the effect of this output on Y. A similar approach would be to attempt a reduction of, or compensation for, these supposed abnormalities in ex-patients, assuming here that there would be ex-patients who continued to exhibit them. The crucial observation in this case would be whether this reduction/compensation would help prevent the subsequent reappearance of symptoms. (The existence of ex-OCD patients who continue to exhibit some brain abnormality would be consistent with that abnormality's playing a role in causing OCD – the elimination of this abnormality might be sufficient, but not necessary, for the alleviation of the disorder.) Points similar to some of the foregoing were raised in Section 6.8.3 as regards the hypothesis that an abnormal thinking style might explain OCD.

The evidence briefly outlined concerning the physical interventions that have been used with OCD might be relevant here. It is debatable whether the surgical interventions used with the disorder reduce, or compensate for, the abnormalities in the basal ganglia and frontal cortex of OCD patients discussed by Rapoport and Wise (1988) and Insel (1988). Although Insel's model, as noted, suggests that these interventions may indeed have such effects, Jenike (1984) argues that the effects of surgical intervention with OCD suggest the involvement of the limbic system in the disorder. The use of clomipramine and other serotonin-reuptake blockers may be more promising for Insel and for Rapoport and Wise, a likely site for the action of these drugs being the basal ganglia, according to Insel and to Rapoport and Wise. Even if this *is* the site of their action, it does not necessarily provide strong evidence that this action reduces, or compensates for, the abnormalities that have been reported there. But such a reduction or compensation might surely be presented in these circumstances (that is, assuming the authors to be correct about the site of the actions of these drugs), as the most *parsimonious* explanation of the anti-OCD effects of these drugs. This explanation would thus be the best available unless the basal ganglia mechanisms on which these drugs acted could be shown both (1) to differ from basal ganglia mechanisms that exhibit abnormalities in OCD patients and (2) not to compensate for those abnormalities when acted on by these drugs. The burden of proof in these circumstances, that is, would rest with those wishing to argue against accounts such as Insel's and Rapoport and Wise's. To the extent that anti-OCD drugs could be shown also to act in the frontal cortex (Rapoport, 1989, p. 68), parsimony may similarly suggest that the best explanation for this action would be the reduction of, or compensation for, the supposed abnormalities reported in this region, too. (Note that Baxter et al., 1987, pp. 215–16) report that some changes in the brains of OCD patients accompany successful drug treatments.)

Even if one could be sure that this reduction of, or compensation for, the reported abnormalities in the brains of OCD patients were the correct explanation of the successful drug treatment of these patients, this would still not be very strong evidence in favour of these abnormalities' playing a role in *producing* OCD. What this finding would show, rather, is that such abnormalities help *maintain* the disorder. The finding that successful drug treatments reduce the rate of relapse among ex-patients would similarly show only that these abnormalities help produce the *reappearance* of the disorder. (Here again the argument follows that of Section 6.8.3 as regards OCD patients and the proposed explanation of their disorder in terms of a hypothesised abnormal thinking style.) To support the claim that these basal ganglia and frontal cortex abnormalities produce, as well as maintain, OCD would require evidence that the *creation* of these abnormalities produces OCD, and this is what the "experiment[s] of nature" (Rapoport, 1989, p. 66) involving patients with Sydenham's chorea, postencephalitic Parkinson's disease and so forth are supposed to suggest. (These "experiments", according to Rapoport, are evidently of more relevance to abnormalities of the basal ganglia than they are to abnormalities of the frontal cortex and thus suggest that the latter may be of less importance in producing OCD.) Suppose, then, that the brain insults involved in these diseases do give rise to OCD symptoms and that the site of these insults is the basal ganglia. These findings would still not be very strong evidence to support the suggestion that these brain insults modelled the supposed abnormalities in OCD patients discussed by Insel and by Rapoport and Wise. Yet it might be argued that parsimony would favour this suggestion – that is, this suggestion would stand as the best explanation available unless it could be shown both that (1) the basal ganglia mechanisms that produced OCD in patients with Sydenham's chorea and other diseases are normal in other OCD patients and that (2) the basal ganglia mechanisms through which Sydenham's chorea and other diseases produce OCD do not have the same effects as any basal ganglia abnormality observed in other OCD patients. (These two possibilities are parallel to those discussed earlier regarding the basal ganglia as a site for the action of anti-OCD drugs.)

It seems, then, that the observations offered by Insel and by Rapoport and Wise, if sound, would indeed support the claim that abnormalities in the basal ganglia, and perhaps also in the frontal cortex, play some role in producing and maintaining OCD.

Rapoport and Wise themselves (1988) offer some reservations about their biological account. They point out that some neurological disorders of the basal ganglia are not associated with OCD and that in at least some cases of those that are, lesions that may be related to the disorder are also found outside the basal ganglia. Rapoport and Wise also note, following Kettl and Marks (1986), that a variety of brain insults with no evident involvement of the basal ganglia can produce OCD. But it may be possible to reconcile these points with the models presented by Rapoport and Wise and by Insel. These models do not require that *all* lesions of the basal ganglia produce OCD; moreover, they make reference, as has been seen, to areas other than the basal ganglia in explaining the disorder. The model is consistent with OCD's being produced by damage to structures that are "downstream from the usual mechanisms that initiate or maintain OCD" (Kettl and Marks, 1986, p. 318) – or indeed by damage to structures that produce OCD by pathways that are entirely separate from those by which the disorder is usually mediated. Grounds for supposing that an abnormality in any brain structure may be among the usual mechanisms that produce and maintain OCD can be provided only by all three of the following: (1) the demonstration that abnormalities in this area can be observed in OCD patients; (2) the demonstration that successful interventions with the disorder are mediated by this area; and (3) evidence that damage to this area produces OCD. (These are the same grounds as those discussed for the role of the basal ganglia and also for the possible role of the frontal cortex.) Note that in category (3), evidence would never, by itself, be sufficient to establish that some brain abnormality is among the usual causes of OCD.

The biological models offered by Rapoport and Wise and by Insel also leave open the possibility that there may be OCD patients who would not exhibit abnormalities such as those discussed by these models, the account of the symptoms of these patients therefore having to be provided in quite other terms. (Indeed, both Luxenberg et al., 1986 [Figure 1, p. 1091] and Baxter et al., 1987 [Figure 1, p. 212; Figures 2 and 3, p. 213; Figure 4, p. 215] report considerable overlaps between their OCD and control groups as regards the variables they examined.)

It was remarked earlier that the origin or origins of the supposed brain abnormalities in OCD patients are worthy of further comment. As previously noted, the observations offered by Rapoport and Wise and by Insel, if sound, support the claim that these abnormalities are not just an effect of OCD, but clearly they tell us little about how these abnormalities *are* to be explained. Indeed, it would be consistent with these observations that these abnormalities are, for example, simply the response of OCD patients to some unusual stress in their environments, a stress that is not shared by other people and that is responsible for producing and maintaining

OCD via these abnormalities. (The association of disorders such as Sydenham's chorea and postencephalitic Parkinson's disease with OCD, in these circumstances, would be explained in terms of these disorders' modelling the effects on the human brain of the unusual stress suffered by OCD patients.) In these circumstances, then, such terms in the foregoing discussion as *abnormality* would need to be used with care – the observed differences between the brains of OCD patients and others would then be a "normal" response to an abnormal environment.

These points are perhaps of only theoretical interest; there are few grounds for believing that the environments of OCD patients contain stresses that are unique to those environments (see, for example, Sections 5.4.3 and 7.6, and Chapter 8). Evidence for the role of genetic factors in OCD (see Section 1.1) may also count against brain abnormalities in OCD patients simply being a response to environmental variables.

7.8   Summary

This chapter has examined a variety of biological findings concerning OCD patients, some proposed animal models of these patients, and a number of the psychological accounts of OCD that have been offered by biological theorists. It has been argued that these biological findings, if sound, would support the claims of authors such as Rapoport and Wise, and Insel, that abnormalities in the basal ganglia, and perhaps also in the frontal cortex, play some role in producing and maintaining OCD; these biological findings have not, however, been subject to either detailed or comprehensive scrutiny here. Claims that the limbic system may also be involved in causing OCD have also been considered, and some possible difficulties for these claims noted. Among the psychological accounts that have been considered in this chapter, Insel's displacement/conflict approach has been suggested as perhaps the most plausible; nonbiological work that may support this approach has been noted.

8   Concluding remarks

8.1   Introduction

The standard diagnostic criteria for OCD have been challenged, and an alternative analysis has been proposed that suggests that no single feature or collection of features is both common and peculiar to all instances of the disorder. Consistent with this position, it was also argued that there is no single way in which OCD may be distinguished either from phobias or from delusional states; and various ways in which OCD may be so distinguished were presented.

The difficulties encountered by the theoretical approaches to OCD that have been reviewed are perhaps more striking than their successes, at least if one attempts to regard any of these approaches as providing a full explanation of the disorder. Nonetheless, *some* of the accounts that have been considered certainly offer observations and suggestions that concern *some* OCD patients and that may well be of importance to any valid account of these patients' psychopathology that eventually emerges. The following observations have been presented as being of possible theoretical importance to an explanation of OCD:

OBSERVATION (1) Evolutionary influences may have a role in selecting the content of some OCD symptoms (stressed by some behavioural writers and some of the Pavlovian personality theorists).

OBSERVATION (2). The basal ganglia (among other possible biological factors) may have a role in producing at least some cases of OCD.

OBSERVATION (3). A neurotic temperament is displayed by many OCD patients (stressed by the Pavlovian personality theorists).

OBSERVATION (4). OCD is co-morbid with certain other disorders (stressed by both the Pavlovian personality theorists and Janet's account).

OBSERVATION (5). Tendencies to timidity and unassertiveness are noted in at least some cases of OCD (stressed by Janet's account, Emmelkamp and van der Heyden's behavioural treatment study, some of the psychodynamic work that was reviewed, and some aspects of the psychological accounts offered on the basis of biological research). The variety of research relevant to this observation will be important to some of the discussion that follows.

The use of exposure with response prevention as a treatment for OCD is argued by a number of theorists (behavioural and otherwise) to be the most important therapeutic advance associated with any of the theoretical approaches discussed, the use of this intervention being associated with the behavioural approach in the sense that it has been most enthusiastically championed by behavioural writers (notwithstanding Pitman's remarks regarding Janet's treatment recommendations). It has been pointed out that debate continues as to the mechanisms by which this intervention may work. Another intervention that is claimed by some writers to be of importance to OCD is clomipramine (and perhaps also other serotonin-reuptake-blocking drugs).

When one brings together the five observations listed at the beginning of this section, the lack of a full explanation for OCD is still evident. Observation (4) suggests that the mechanisms that produce OCD overlap to some extent with those that produce certain other disorders; observations (3) and (5) may provide examples of such mechanisms. Observations (3) and (5) thus feature characteristics that appear in conjunction with disorders other than OCD and are insufficient to account for such features as the bizarre thinking, failures of memory concerning everyday actions and repetitive behavior that are reported by OCD patients. A full account of OCD would need to go further; it would have to provide details not only of the mechanisms that OCD shares with other disorders, but also of those that are specific to OCD (or perhaps of those *combinations* that are, if none of the mechanisms that make up any such combination(s) turned out to be unique to the disorder). Further research into the proposed evolutionary influences of observation (1) is unlikely to furnish us with such details and thus looks as if it will be unable to provide us – in conjunction with observations such as (3), (4) and (5) – with a full account of OCD. As argued earlier, evolutionary influences such as those previously discussed do not appear to be at all relevant to many OCD symptoms and, in the case of those symptom contents that perhaps are of evolutionary significance, these hypothesised influences tend to be poor at accounting for the very features that observations (3), (4) and (5) also have difficulty explaining (see Section 3.5).

What about observation (2) – the possible role in OCD of the basal ganglia (among other biological factors)? Biological findings relevant to OCD have received neither detailed nor comprehensive scrutiny in the foregoing chapters. Nonetheless, it may be that research along these lines is very promising as regards the possibility that a complete account of OCD will eventually be provided. Thus, at present, one cannot rule out the possibility that there is little difference between the various experiences that may help to produce OCD and the experiences that may help to produce at least some of the other conditions that feature in observation (4); genetic contributions to OCD and these other conditions may also overlap to some extent (see Section 1.1). It may turn out to be the case, then, that one can only begin to make sense of why, for example, one person develops OCD, and another agoraphobia, when one considers such factors as biological differences between these people that are of genetic origin. (Observation [4] would suggest that these different biological characteristics could also co-occur, of course.) Whether or not biological factors can play this role in explaining OCD and, if this is the case, whether or not those factors that have been identified in existing biological research will be among those that do so, remain questions for further research. (That some of the existing biological findings have been poorly controlled, as noted in Sections 7.2 and 7.3, may clearly be of importance in this context.)

De Silva (1988) suggests that "the limited progress that has been made in our understanding" (p. 195) of OCD may be partly due to "the tendency...to assume that [OCD represents] a unitary phenomenon with each theoretical model being offered to account for a diversity of symptoms and presentations" (pp. 202–203). De Silva argues that this attempt to adopt a "unitary" approach may be mistaken and suggests one or two phenomenological distinctions that, he argues, may be important from the point of view of the explanation of OCD. Yet the importance of any phenomenological distinction to the explanation and/or treatment of OCD remains an open question. It may be that there are no important subdivisions of OCD from the point of view of explanation or treatment, or (perhaps more plausibly) that such subdivisions do not correspond to any differences in the kind of symptoms reported. Insel (1982) suggests one such subdivision based on the *age of onset* of the disorder; another subdivision, concerning the patient's level of assertiveness rather than the nature of his or her symptoms, was discussed in Section 4.7.3 and will be further examined.

Possible lines for future research regarding many of the theoretical approaches considered in the foregoing chapters have been noted. Can one bring at least some of these possibilities together and thus point out further research that would be informed by several different approaches to OCD? This would certainly be no guarantee that such research would be more promising than other work not so informed. However, the point (or points) at which different lines of inquiry converge should provide a reasonable starting point (or starting points) for further work; at this point (or at these points), arguments within any given one of the converging lines of inquiry may be able both to provide independent support for arguments from these other lines of inquiry and similarly to receive such support from those arguments.

The discussion in the remainder of this chapter will take the following course. Before the discussion of an example of various lines of research from the foregoing chapters that are in some respects converging, some attempt will be made briefly to clarify what counts as progress in scientific research and critically discuss an example of what Eysenck (1977) has presented as such progress in the case of OCD. An example of some converging lines of evidence will then be discussed at some length, and an attempt made to determine whether or not these converging lines of evidence may be said to amount to "progressive" research. The lines of evidence chosen for this examination are those listed under observation (5); this is not, of course, to deny that there may be other examples of such convergence in the work reviewed in the foregoing chapters.

8.2   Progress in scientific research

What, then, would it mean for any of the work that has been reviewed in the foregoing chapters to be *progressive scientific research*, as these terms would be understood by contemporary philosophers of science? Lakatos (1970) distinguishes between *progressive* and *degenerating* scientific research. On Lakatos's account, research is *theoretically progressive* if it leads to new predictions, and *empirically progressive* if these predictions are successful. *Degenerating* scientific research, in contrast, is described by Lakatos as being that which is yielding neither new predictions nor empirical successes. Such research will also have had its former empirical successes (if any) accounted for by some rival approach, and this rival approach, on Lakatos's account, will have had empirical successes of its own that the degenerating approach will only be able to explain by resorting to ad hoc manoeuvres (Gholson and Barker, 1985). Putnam (1974) provides an important qualification of Lakatos's view when he suggests that the success of a scientific theory may consist in the elegant or striking explanation of some *already known* fact instead of (or as well as) the correct prediction of some novel finding. Similarly, what is important about a theory is surely not that it leads to *new* predictions and findings, but rather that these predictions and findings are such that rival theories cannot *plausibly explain* them. This point will prove to be of importance to the discussion that follows and may be implicit in Lakatos's further suggestion that the predictions made by progressive research should be "stunning" (Lakatos, 1970).

Putnam believes himself to be giving an account of Kuhn's (1962) notion of a paradigm in his aforementioned remarks, whereas Lakatos (1970), on the basis of his criticisms of Kuhn's work, is stating the conditions for progress in what he describes as a "research programme" (that is, a succession of theories linked by a common core of shared ideas, this core itself not being open to immediate empirical refutation; see Lauden, 1977, for some criticisms of Lakatos's position). It is unclear whether any of the work on OCD described in the foregoing chapters is substantial enough to be regarded as either a paradigm or a research programme. At the risk of misusing the ideas of Lakatos and Putnam, however, let us suspend judgment here as to whether any of this work could be so regarded and ask only if any of the accounts of OCD presented may be said to be progressive, insofar as they have produced a better explanation of existing observations than have alternative approaches and/or have predicted some novel finding that these other approaches would have difficulty in making sense of.

Before doing this, it should be noted that, according to some writers, it may be a mistake to judge some of the work that was reviewed in the foregoing chapters in these terms at all, particularly the psychodynamic work reviewed in Chapter 5. On this view, there is a fundamental difference between the understanding of behaviour in terms of higher-level psychological processes (such as intentions, beliefs, desires) and the explanation of phenomena in the natural sciences (Ryle, 1949; Anscombe, 1957; Melden, 1961), and it is argued that these higher-level processes cannot be part of any scientific explanation. Jaspers (1963) similarly contrasts the understanding of "meaningful connections", on the one hand, and of causal explanation, on the other. Drawing on Jaspers's account, Bolton (1984) suggests, that one of the other contrasts between meaningful connections and causal connections is that the former are particular, the latter general. In the case of meaningful connections, that is, it is suggested that generalisations across individuals and individual conditions result in a loss of information, whereas in the natural sciences, generalisations are "complete summaries of the data inherent in particular instances" (Bolton, 1984, p. 755). (Related to this point, the importance of the details of individual cases to psychodynamic work has already been noted in Section 5.1.)

A full discussion of this position is not being offered here, but it would surely be implausible to argue on philosophical grounds such as these alone that there are *no* useful generalisations concerning higher-level psychological processes in OCD patients or in subgroups of such patients. These generalisations would themselves have to be subject to individual scrutiny before it could be decided whether or not this is so, and this scrutiny, it might be argued, should include the examination of these generalisations in the terms provided by Lakatos, Putnam and others.

Other contrasts Jaspers draws between meaningful and causal connections are that the former are apprehended in a more immediate manner than the latter and that the insight provided by the understanding of meaningful connections is distinct from that provided by the scientific investigation of causal relationships. These points are critically discussed by Cooper and Cooper (1983); also see Davidson (1980, especially Essays 1–5) and Woodfield (1976).

It is argued by Eysenck (1977) that the behavioural approach to OCD is *progressive,* in the terms of Lakatos's work, and Eysenck specifically cites in defence of this claim the results of exposure with response prevention in the treatment of the disorder. He argues that these results provide a stunning, or at least psychiatrically important, confirmation of a prediction made by the behavioural approach.

Against the suggestion that this confirmation makes the behavioural approach progressive, and leaving to one side the question of the efficacy of exposure with response prevention, there are various alternative explanations available as to why this intervention might help some OCD patients. Gray (1979, 1982), for example, has put forward an innate fear account of OCD (see Section 3.5). Although this account meets with difficulties of its own, it is able to explain both the treatment results Eysenck cites in favour of the behavioural approach, as well as a number of further findings that can be dealt with by that approach only by the introduction of ad hoc manoeuvres – for example, Eysenck's explanation in terms of his notion that the incubation of fear-eliciting stimuli does not undergo extinction (see Section 2.2). This suggests, then, that contrary to Eysenck's position, the behavioural account of OCD is at present degenerating, in Lakatos's sense of this term.

There are, furthermore, still other accounts of the mechanisms by which exposure with response prevention may help some OCD patients, accounts that may be derived from still other proposed explanations of OCD – for example, explanations in terms of the poor spontaneous structuring of experience (see Section 6.7), in terms of low perceived self-efficacy, and in terms of psychodynamic mechanisms. Thus, in the case of this last explanation, it might be suggested that preventing compulsive behaviour from being carried out deprives the patient of his or her defence mechanisms, bringing about a therapeutic confrontation with the "hidden feeling", to use Malan's terminology (see Section 5.4.2). This may, then, suggest the manner in which a psychodynamic account such as Malan's (1979) would attempt to explain why exposure with response prevention should be a successful intervention with some OCD patients, a task that Malan himself suggests to be important for such an account; Janet's account of this success would perhaps most plausibly be along similar lines (also see Section 4.7.3). Certain aspects of some clinical reports, furthermore, appear to be consistent with this account of the action of exposure with response prevention (Jakes, 1992, pp. 276–7).

Exposure with response prevention is open to a variety of explanations because it targets the contents of the patient's symptoms. Clearly, *any* account must acknowledge these contents to be part of the patient's problem (in the trivial sense that they are what the symptoms consist of), and any account is thus likely to be able to offer *some* reason why this type of therapy might be of use.

8.3   OCD and assertiveness

Can an example be provided, then, from among the theoretical approaches to OCD discussed in the foregoing chapters, of some ideas concerning the disorder that are shared by a number of these theoretical approaches, and that, although being far from providing a complete account of OCD, are progressive, in the sense outlined in Section 8.2? One example, already noted in Section 8.1, will be considered. It was pointed out in connection both with Janet's discussion of OCD (see Chapter 4) and with the psychodynamic work discussed in Chapter 5, that a tendency to unassertiveness is observed in some OCD patients. Janet (1903) and Malan (1979) suggest that a failure to act assertively and/or to express aggressive feelings may help precipitate the symptoms of some OCD patients and that these symptoms may, therefore, be alleviated by an intervention that successfully encourages these patients to behave more assertively and/or to express their aggressive feelings to a greater extent. Emmelkamp and van der Heyden (1980), in reporting a behavioural intervention with OCD patients, make exactly the same suggestions, and some aspects of the psychological accounts offered on the basis of biological research into the disorder also overlap to some extent with these ideas (for example, Insel's remarks regarding the role of conflict and aggressiveness in OCD [see Section 7.6]; Claridge [1985] also offers a few suggestions along these lines [see Section 3.7.2], although he does so only when he himself tries to draw together various lines of investigation concerning OCD). An attempt will be made to show that these suggestions are theoretically progressive – that is, that they offer explanations and predictions that cannot readily be supported by approaches that do not make use of the ideas shared by Janet, Emmelkamp and van der Heyden, Malan and so forth. This will be followed by a few remarks as to whether these suggestions may also be regarded as empirically progressive.

Assertion training is an intervention that encourages patients to behave more assertively and/or to express their aggressive feelings to a greater extent (Emmelkamp and van der Heyden, 1980). Emmelkamp and van der Heyden's position, and those aspects of Janet's and Malan's accounts that coincide with that position, would predict that this intervention should help to reduce the symptoms of at least some OCD patients. Can it be shown, then, that in contrast to the success claimed for exposure with response prevention, this prediction is a difficult one for other accounts of OCD to make? Can one argue, that is, that a favourable response of patients to this intervention would indeed be likely to result from its increasing their level of assertiveness in the manner suggested by Emmelkamp and van der Heyden, for example, rather than from its being related to mechanisms that could be more easily accommodated within accounts of OCD that make no reference to unassertive behaviour or unexpressed aggressive feelings as precipitants of some OCD symptoms? This demonstration is central to the question of whether Emmelkamp and van der Heyden's account and, again, those aspects of Janet's and Malan's with which that account overlaps, may be said to be in the present respect theoretically progressive, and it is consideration of this question that will be the focus of the bulk of the following discussion. A further question concerns the extent to that there is any evidence for this prediction's being correct, and a few remarks concerning the little evidence available will also be offered.

8.4 Alternative bases for the prediction that assertion training may help some OCD patients

8.4.1 Introduction

How else, then, might this prediction be supported other than in the terms offered by the overlapping aspects of accounts such as Emmelkamp and van der Heyden's, Janet's, or Malan's? Are there not alternative explanations of the mechanisms by which an assertion training intervention might help some cases of OCD, explanations that are consistent with other accounts of these cases? Several such alternative bases for the prediction that assertion training should help some OCD patients will now be considered. (Reed's suggestion that his account would be unable to support this prediction has already been briefly considered; see Sections 6.1.2 and 6.7.)

8.4.2 Boyd and Levis's work

Boyd and Levis (1983) offer a number of points that arise specifically in connection with the study conducted by Emmelkamp and van der Heyden (1980), which was discussed in Section 4.7.3. Boyd and Levis draw attention to the fact that Emmelkamp and van der Heyden have been dealing with obsessions in which the contents involve the theme of hurting other people. Boyd and Levis correctly point out that, for such cases of OCD, contact with the people whom the patient fears he or she may harm (as would be required by assertion training exercises) could be operating via the same mechanisms as those involved in exposure with response prevention to produce the therapeutic effects reported. And as argued, the therapeutic success of exposure with response prevention is probably consistent with many of the theoretical approaches to OCD considered in the foregoing chapters – on Boyd and Levis's interpretation, in other words, many of these approaches would probably also be able to make Emmelkamp and van der Heyden's prediction.

A powerful test of this interpretation would be to treat with assertion training patients whose symptom contents do not involve contact with other people at all. It should be possible to carry out such a test. Emmelkamp and van der Heyden (1980, p. 29) suggest that "research into the treatment of obsessions should take into account the differences in the content of various obsessions", and thus they make their case for using assertion training specifically with harming obsessions. Clinical experience, however, suggests that this claim may place too much emphasis on symptom content as an indicator of the nature of the patient's difficulties. Indeed, Emmelkamp himself (1982, p. 238) makes this point. Thus, patients whose problems concern, for example, checking plug sockets or cleaning their hands, sometimes report that difficulties in asserting themselves are an important precipitant of their obsessions. Emmelkamp and van der Heyden's prediction, applied to the use of assertion training in the treatment of patients such as these, would not encounter Boyd and Levis's objection.

It is important to note that Boyd and Levis's approach cannot readily explain, for example, several of Emmelkamp and van der Heyden's observations that may be used to support the prediction that assertion training may help some OCD patients. Thus, Emmelkamp and van der Heyden's observations that their patients were unassertive prior to therapy and that some of these patients had their obsessions provoked by situations that required them to be in some measure assertive, are both used by Emmelkamp and van der Heyden to support their prediction, but they are not explained by Boyd and Levis's position. Therefore, to the extent that these observations may be replicated (and Janet and some of the psychodynamic approaches considered earlier offer similar observations), any alternative basis for the prediction offered by Emmelkamp and van der Heyden should be able to make sense of them.

It is also worth noting that Boyd and Levis's explanation would probably differ from Emmelkamp and van der Heyden's in its implications for the experience of the subject taking part in assertion training exercises. Boyd and Levis's hypothesis suggests that these subjects would experience their obsessions early on in such exercises, these obsessions gradually reducing both within and between sessions, as a result of exposure to provoking cues during the assertion exercises. Emmelkamp and van der Heyden's account probably has contrasting predictions. If obsessions are, as these authors say, the result of such situations as the patient's failing to deal appropriately with criticism, and if assertion exercises involve the patient's dealing more successfully with such situations, then on this hypothesis the obsessions will most likely not occur at all during these exercises, or will at most occur only in a milder form.

8.4.3 Another exposure-based account?

A different approach to that of Boyd and Levis leads to the apparently similar prediction that assertion training should help some OCD patients but should do so by means of exposure mechanisms. This approach, like that of Boyd and Levis, may appear to suggest that various theoretical approaches are consistent with this prediction. This approach would argue that what the patient is exposed to in such training is the consequences of asserting himself. The patient, according to this approach, should discover in assertion training that it is, for example, possible to refuse the demands of others, or to make reasonable demands of them, without spoiling all subsequent contact with them.

But to describe the foregoing as an exposure-based account of how assertion training might work is misleading. The account clearly shares much in common with the grounds on which Emmelkamp and van der Heyden, Janet and Malan would make the same prediction; in particular, like those approaches, it makes the crucial anti-exposure suggestion that patients will not be helped in assertion training by being *brought into contact with the contents of their symptoms*. (These contents involve the theme of harming others by attacking or insulting them, for example, not by making or refusing demands in an appropriate manner.) The account is thus best regarded, despite appearances, as a restatement of Emmelkamp and van der Heyden's own position (and a restatement of the relevant aspects of Janet's and Malan's accounts) as regards the mechanisms by which assertion training might work.

8.4.4 Assertive behaviour as reciprocal inhibition

Wolpe (1958) proposes another basis for the prediction that assertion training should be of some therapeutic value (as applied, in this case, to anxiety disorders in general, rather than specifically to OCD). This prediction in supported by Wolpe in terms of "reciprocal inhibition". Assertive behaviour should serve to reduce anxiety by being incompatible with it, he suggests, in much the same way that, for example, relaxation exercises, sexual arousal or feeding would also be held by Wolpe to reduce anxiety. This proposal, if correct, would suggest that any success that assertion training might be shown to have in treating OCD is perhaps consistent with a variety of different approaches to OCD and is certainly consistent with the behavioural account (see Chapter 2) to which Wolpe himself subscribes.

Like Boyd and Levis's approach, however, Wolpe's account fails to make sense of the wider picture of unassertive behaviour's leading to the appearance of symptoms prior to treatment. Therefore, to the extent that this wider picture obtains among OCD patients, Wolpe's account, as a basis for the prediction that assertion training should help some such patients, is less convincing than are the overlapping aspects of the accounts offered by Emmelkamp and van der Heyden, Janet, and Malan.

8.4.5 Assertive behaviour and perceived self-efficacy

Yet another alternative explanation might make better sense of this wider picture. Bandura (1978) argues that a wide range of anxiety disorders, including OCD and phobias, result from the patient's belief that he is unable to cope with whatever it is that he fears – the patient, to use Bandura's phrase, has "low perceived self-efficacy" as regards the stimuli and situations he fears. Bandura also argues that all behavioural treatments work by increasing "perceptions of self-efficacy". Bandura would suggest, for example, both that a social phobic's fundamental problem is his belief that he is unable to deal with social situations, and that exposure with response prevention works with such a patient by enabling him to discover that he can deal with such situations and/or by enabling him to acquire some means by which to do so. Bandura suggests that the "increased perceptions of self-efficacy" this produces may generalise, leading to improvements elsewhere in the patient's functioning – for example, regarding his suffering from fears with entirely unrelated contents.

Applying Bandura's approach to assertion training, one can argue that this intervention, if successful, will cause an increase in the perceptions of self-efficacy of patients as regards their interaction with other people. Furthermore, any improvement in the obsessions of patients such as Emmelkamp and van der Heyden's as a result of assertion training would be seen by this approach to be due to the generalisation of these increased perceptions of self-efficacy to the patients' symptom areas, in a manner similar to that in which, Bandura argues, such perceptions sometimes generalise from one phobia to another. The cognitive-behavioural account (see Section 2.8) might be able to offer a somewhat similar basis for Emmelkamp and van der Heyden's prediction.

A full evaluation of Bandura's self-efficacy hypothesis is beyond the scope of the present discussion, but a few points regarding this approach are worth noting. The support provided by the self-efficacy theory for the prediction that assertion training should help some OCD patients, unlike Boyd and Levis's and that taken from Wolpe's work, does not take issue with Emmelkamp and van der Heyden's claim that assertion training should reduce OCD via its effects on the low level of assertiveness of some patients. Nonetheless, this interpretation does question the mechanisms that Emmelkamp and van der Heyden suggest bring about this effect; therefore, one may use this interpretation to deny the role that Emmelkamp and van der Heyden assign to unexpressed aggressive feelings in producing some obsessions in the first place.

It should be noted that this perceived self-efficacy approach, being itself yet another account of OCD (and other psychopathology), probably does not provide a means by which most of the other accounts of OCD reviewed in the foregoing chapters can be reconciled with the prediction that assertion training should help some OCD patients (with the possible exception, as noted, of the cognitive-behavioural account). But there are a number of difficulties facing this application of the perceived–self-efficacy account. It is probably too ambitious to attempt to support Emmelkamp and van der Heyden's prediction in exactly the same terms as those in which Bandura already tries to explain such a wide range of other phenomena. Emmelkamp and his colleagues, for example, have also used assertion training with agoraphobics (Emmelkamp et al., 1983) and found that improvements in the assertiveness of these patients tended to occur independently of any changes in their symptoms (although see Emmelkamp, 1982, p. 127). How, then, could Bandura's approach predict that the hypothesised improvement in perceptions of self-efficacy should generalise from the patient's increased assertiveness to symptom contents in the case of harming obsessions, given that it fails to do so in the case of agoraphobia? The unitary explanation of these different disorders and their treatment in terms of perceptions of self-efficacy is probably silent as to this question – a question that does not arise for Emmelkamp and van der Heyden's more specific account from which no prediction as to the effects of using assertion training with agoraphobics can be derived. It is, furthermore, difficult to see how some harming obsessions could be the result of perceptions of low self-efficacy and why, therefore, they should be eliminated by any hypothesised increase in such perceptions. What, for example, would such an account make of the impulse to harm others? (Note, in particular, that such a symptom is not a doubt that one may have harmed others, which could perhaps be represented as low perceived self-efficacy as regards one's self-control.) Perhaps the account would suggest that distress results not from the impulse per se, but from the patient's low perceived self-efficacy regarding his ability to hold the impulse under control. This renders the account a little like some of the suggestions offered by Salkovskis (1985, 1989) as regards OCD in general; objections to these suggestions have already been offered elsewhere (see Section 2.8 and Jakes, 1989a, 1989b). Perhaps doubts that one may have harmed others might be argued instead to produce the impulse to act in this manner, as Gray (1982) has suggested. But there is nothing in Bandura's perceived–self-efficacy account that would explain why this should be so, and the account within which Gray himself makes this suggestion has been criticised earlier (see Section 3.6).

8.4.6 Conclusion

Four alternative bases for the prediction that assertion training should help some OCD patients have now been considered. Three of these bases would have been consistent with explanations other than those offered by the overlapping aspects of the accounts of Emmelkamp and van der Heyden, Janet, and Malan of how OCD arises. It has been suggested, however, that all three of these bases are probably less plausible than the position defended by Emmelkamp and van der Heyden (although this position faces difficulties of its own, as discussed later), and the remaining alternative turns out, on examination, to be a restatement of their position. The present discussion provides, therefore, some support for the suggestion that the successful use of assertion training with some cases of OCD cannot be plausibly explained by many of the various alternative approaches to the disorder. To this extent, therefore, Emmelkamp and van der Heyden's position, and those aspects of Janet's and Malan's accounts that coincide with it, have been shown to be theoretically progressive – they lead, that is, to a prediction that cannot be as strongly supported by the other accounts that have been considered here. It is probably also the case, therefore, that assertion training can in this respect be contrasted with exposure with response prevention (see Section 8.2), although it of course remains to be seen whether hypotheses other than those considered here could support Emmelkamp and van der Heyden's prediction.

8.5   Evidence that confirms the prediction that assertiveness training may help some OCD patients

The prediction that assertiveness training may help some OCD patients has not been well researched, and indeed the only controlled study that addresses it appears to be the one by Emmelkamp and van der Heyden that has already been referred to (see Section 4.7.3). Emmelkamp (1982, p. 220) remarks that it is "astonishing" how little controlled work has been carried out on OCD patients in this regard, despite Wolpe's (1958) early suggestion that assertion training might be a useful intervention for these patients; Emmelkamp (1982, pp. 219–21) presents two case studies in which assertion training appears to produce clinically significant improvements.

It seems, then, appropriate to consider in a little more detail here exactly what the findings of Emmelkamp and van der Heyden's (1980) study were. These authors compared the effects of assertion training and of thought stopping as treatments for harming obsessions. To do this, a crossover design was employed, enabling the comparison of these two treatments to be made both within and between subjects. Six patients, all women, were included in the study, half receiving thought stopping prior to assertion training, half receiving these two treatments in the reverse order.

Emmelkamp and van der Heyden's statements regarding the outcome of their study are in some measure equivocal, but the authors report that "assertiveness training led to a...reduction of the frequency of obsessions for most patients" (p. 33) and state that "most patients seemed to have benefitted more from assertiveness training than from thought stopping" (p. 28). The justification for these claims as to the superiority of assertion training is that it led to a reduction in the frequency of obsessions in at least four (and probably five) cases, whereas improvement occurred after the administration of thought stopping in only two cases. One may evidently conclude that there is some, although by no means conclusive, support here for Emmelkamp and van der Heyden's remarks concerning the results of assertion training with their OCD patients.

Assertion training also led to a significant increase in assertive behaviour, Emmelkamp and van der Heyden report. This was despite the fact that assertiveness scores at the pretreatment stage were artificially high because of two patients who were "scoring within normal ranges" of assertiveness at this stage due to "a lack of insight into their interpersonal problems" (p. 33).

Emmelkamp and van der Heyden's study plainly has a number of important shortcomings that should be borne in mind when considering its findings. As noted, only six patients were included, and each of these received both assertion training and thought stopping. This design, as Emmelkamp and van der Heyden themselves point out, is only able to answer questions about short-term therapeutic effects – a between-group study would be required to assess the long-term effectiveness of either intervention (although see Emmelkamp, 1982, for follow-up data on some of these patients).

The use of larger numbers of patients should be made possible by something that was pointed out earlier (see Section 6.7) – Emmelkamp and van der Heyden have probably taken symptom content as too important an indicator of underlying pathology, and it may therefore be possible, by means of this intervention, to help OCD patients other than those with harming obsessions. Of equal importance, and as noted earlier (for example, Section 4.5.2), some OCD patients are *overassertive* and *rigid* in their dealings with others, precisely the opposite profile to that observed among Emmelkamp and van der Heyden's patients. This wider profile of the patient's level of assertiveness – not the nature of his or her symptom contents – may be the most important indicator of the likely value of assertion training for him or her (this point calling to mind the suggestion in Section 8.1 that the most important subdivisions of OCD may not have to do with phenomenology or symptom types at all).

Emmelkamp and van der Heyden's study would also have been improved by assertion training's being compared with a more established treatment than thought stopping. Their conclusion that most patients seem to have benefitted more from assertion training than from thought stopping in itself tells us little as to the value of assertion training, given the uncertain status of thought stopping; at most, this entitles one to conclude that assertion training is more effective than an alternative that might have some face validity for the patient but is not a well-established treatment for OCD (Emmelkamp, 1982, pp. 228–9). One may conclude that it has not been convincingly shown that the account of OCD advanced by Emmelkamp and van der Heyden, and those aspects of Janet's and Malan's formulations that overlap with it, are at present empirically progressive (as defined in Section 8.1) as regards their prediction that assertion training should be an effective treatment for OCD.

8.6 Further points and questions raised by Emmelkamp and van der Heyden's study

There are a number of further issues worth noting. Emmelkamp and van der Heyden's study has the virtue of attempting to *manipulate* (with assertion training) a variable (the unassertiveness of the patients suffering harming obsessions) that these authors hypothesise to be contributing to the production of these obsessions in order to see if these obsessions are reduced by this manipulation. It is thus possible to test Emmelkamp and van der Heyden's account (and those aspects of Janet's and Malan's accounts that overlap with it) with more than just correlational or observational evidence. There is a regrettable absence of data of this kind for some of the approaches to OCD considered earlier, as was particularly noted in connection with Reed's account (see Section 6.8.3).

 Emmelkamp and van der Heyden's account also raises the question of whether the precipitants of some cases of OCD are primarily interpersonal in nature. The successful use of assertion training for such cases would not demonstrate that the precipitants are primarily interpersonal; it would suggest interpersonal factors to be *an* important precipitant of some cases of OCD, but it would not show such factors to be of overriding importance. For example, an alternative position might suggest that situations in which these patients are required to assert themselves are simply highly anxiety provoking for them, and this precipitates the symptoms of these patients. This view would argue that these patients would be similarly affected by sources of anxiety not involving assertion or social interaction at all (for example, anticipating surgery or dental treatment). Emmelkamp and van der Heyden suggest that the *contents* of harming obsessions indicate that anger is playing an important role in producing such obsessions, but symptom content can in itself surely not provide a conclusive argument for this (also see Section 4.5.5); in any event, it seems, as previously argued, that not all of the obsessions provoked by the inappropriately unassertive behaviour of patients are harming obsessions.

 This is an area that is suitable for further research, with two related issues standing in need of investigation. The first of these is the extent to which interpersonal difficulties are the most important precipitants of distress in some OCD sufferers; the second is the nature of the most important precipitating mood disturbance for those patients whose symptoms are provoked by interpersonal situations – and, in particular, whether this mood disturbance involves anxiety, anger or some combination of these, and whether still further types of mood disturbance are also involved (for example, depression and guilt). The literature on the nature of the mood disturbance among OCD patients in general has yet to provide a definitive answer to these questions (for example, Beech and Liddell, 1974; Rachman and Hodgson, 1980; Reed, 1985), and one is entitled to conclude that the hypothesis of unexpressed aggressive feelings' precipitating some obsessions is at present even less well supported than is the rather less specific suggestion that it is unassertive behaviour in certain situations that precipitates these obsessions. Further phenomenological work is needed in order to support hypotheses that specify unexpressed aggressive feelings or anger, and/or still other forms of distress (such as guilt at such feelings, as Emmelkamp and van der Heyden also suggest) to be the primary emotional disturbances in such cases.

8.7   Final comment

For no want of effort, the discussion of the foregoing chapters has produced no definitive account of OCD. It is, of course, rather ironic that a book on the present topic should have examined so many attempts to arrive at certainty, only for these attempts to have largely collapsed in doubts. Still, if it is the case that "the best lack all conviction", OCD will at least be distinguished by its more diligent researchers' sharing this characteristic with many of those whom their research concerns. And one should, in having no full account of the disorder, be in good company.

References

Adler A 1964 Compulsion Neurosis. In: Ansbacher HL, Ansbacher RR (Eds) Superiority and Social Interest. Northwestern University Press, Evanston, Ill.

Akhtar S, Wig NN, Varma VK, Pershad D, Verma SK 1975 A phenomenological analysis of symptoms in obsessive-compulsive neurosis. British Journal of Psychiatry 127: 342–348

American Psychiatric Association (1980) Diagnostic and Statistical Manual of Mental Disorders, 3rd edition. APA, Washington

  (1987) Diagnostic and Statistical Manual of Mental Disorders, 3rd edition, revised. APA, Washington

  (1994) Diagnostic and Statistical Manual of Mental Disorders, 4th edition. APA, Washington

Anscombe GEM 1957 Intention. Basil Blackwell, Oxford

Anthony JC, Folstein M, Romanoski AJ et al 1985 Comparison of lay diagnostic interview schedule and a standardized psychiatric diagnosis: experience in Eastern Baltimore, Archives of General Psychiatry 42: 667–675

Bandura A 1978 Self-efficacy: towards a unifying theory of behavioural change. Advances in Behaviour Research and Therapy 1: 139–161

Bartlett FC 1932 Remembering: A Study in Experimental and Social Psychology. Cambridge University Press, Cambridge

Baxter LR, Phelps ME, Mazziotta JC, Guze BH, Schwartz JM, Setion CE 1987 Local cerebral glucose metabolic rates in obsessive-compulsive disorder. Archives of General Psychiatry 44: 211–216

Bebbington P 1990 The prevalence of obsessive compulsive disorder in the general population. Paper presented at the Duphar National Symposium on Obsessive Compulsive Disorder, London

Beck AT 1976 Cognitive Therapy and the Emotional Disorders. International Universities Press, New York

Beck AT, Emery G, Greenberg RL 1985 Anxiety Disorders and Phobias: A Cognitive Perspective. Basic Books, New York

Beck AT, Ward CH, Mendelson M, Mock JE, Erbaugh JK 1961 An inventory for measuring depression. Archives of General Psychiatry 4: 561–571

Beech HR 1971 Ritualistic activity in obsessional patients. Journal of Psychosomatic Research 15: 417–422

  1974 (Ed) Obsessional States. Methuen, London

Beech HR, Liddell A 1974 Decision-making, mood states and ritualistic behaviour among obsessional patients. In: Beech HR (Ed) Obsessional States. Methuen, London

Beech HR, Perigault J 1974 Towards a theory of obsessional disorder. In: Beech HR (Ed) Obsessional States. Methuen, London

166

Bersch PJ 1980 Eysenck's theory of incubation: a critical analysis. Behaviour Research and Therapy 18: 11–17

Black A 1974 The natural history of obsessional disorders. In: Beech HR (Ed) Obsessional States. Methuen, London

Bolton D 1984 Philosophy and psychiatry. In: McGuffin P, Shanks MF, Hodgson RJ (Eds) The Scientific Principles of Psychopathology. Academic Press, London

Boyd TL, Levis DJ 1983 Exposure is a necessary condition for fear reduction: a reply to de Silva and Rachman. Behaviour Research and Therapy 21: 143–149

Broadbent DE, Broadbent MHP, Jones JL 1986 Performance correlates of self-reported cognitive failure and of obsessionality. British Journal of Clinical Psychology 25: 285–299

Carey G, Gottesman II 1981 Twin and family studies of anxiety, phobic and obsessive disorders. In: Klein DF, Rabkin J (Eds) Anxiety: New Research and Changing Concepts. Raven, New York

Carr A 1974 Compulsive neurosis: a review of the literature. Psychological Bulletin 81: 311–318

Claridge GS 1985 The Origins of Mental Illness. Basil Blackwell, Oxford

Cobb J 1986 Behavioural/psychological treatment of generalised anxiety. Unpublished paper

Cooper PJ, Cooper Z 1985 A note on explanation and understanding in psychology. British Journal of Medical Psychology 58: 19–24

Cooper Z, Cooper PJ 1988 Classification and diagnosis. In: Miller E, Cooper PJ (Eds) Adult Abnormal Psychology. Churchill Livingstone, Edinburgh, London, Melbourne, and New York

Cottraux J 1990 Exposure in combination with drug therapy. Paper presented at the Duphar National Symposium on Obsessive Compulsive Disorder, London

Cummings JL, Frankel M 1985 Gilles de la Tourette's syndrome and the neurological basis of obsessions and compulsions. Biological Psychiatry 20: 1117–1126

Davidson D 1980 Essays on Actions and Events. Clarendon Press, Oxford

DSM-III: see American Psychiatric Association (1980)

DSM-III-R: see American Psychiatric Association (1987)

DSM-IV: see American Psychiatric Association (1994)

Eaton WW, Kramer M, Anthony JC, Dryman A, Shapiro S, Locke BZ 1989 The incidence of specific DIS/DSM III mental disorders: data from NIMH Epidemiologic Catchment Area Program. Acta Psychiatrica Scandinavica 79: 163–178

Edwards W 1982 Conservatism in human information processing. In: Kahneman D, Slovic P, Tversky A (Eds) Judgement under Uncertainty: Heuristics and Biases. Cambridge University Press, Cambridge

Emmelkamp PMG 1982 Phobic and Obsessive-Compulsive Disorders: Theory, Research and Practice. Plenum, New York

Emmelkamp PMG and van der Heyden H 1980 The treatment of harming obsessions. Behavioural Analysis and Modification 4: 28–35

Emmelkamp PMG, van der Hout A, de Vries K 1983 Assertive training for agoraphobics. Behaviour Research and Therapy 21: 63–68

England SL, Dickerson M 1988 Intrusive thoughts: unpleasantness not the major cause of uncontrollability. Behaviour Research and Therapy 26: 277–279

Eysenck HJ 1952 The Scientific Study of Personality. Routledge and Kegan Paul, London

1977 Behaviour therapy: dogma or applied science? In: Feldman MP and Broadhurst A Theoretical and Experimental Bases of the Behaviour Therapies. Wiley, London

1979 The conditioning model of neurosis. Behavioural and Brain Sciences 2: 155–166

Eysenck HJ, Eysenck SBG 1964 Manual of the Eysenck Personality Inventory. University of London Press, London

1975 Manual of the Eysenck Personality Questionnaire. Hodder and Stroughton, London

Eysenck HJ, Rachman SJ 1965 The Causes and Cures of Neuroses. Routledge and Kegan Paul, London

Fenichel O 1977 The Psychoanalytic Theory of Neurosis. Norton, New York

Ferenczi S 1980 Stages in the development of the sense of reality. In: First Contributions to Psycho-analysis. Authorized translation by E. Jones. New York, Brunner/Mazel

Fineberg N 1990 OCD and depression: similarities and differences. Paper presented at the Duphar National Symposium on Obsessive-Compulsive Disorder, London

Fish F 1968 The varieties of delusion. International Journal of Psychiatry 6: No 1

Foa EB, Steketee G, Ozarow BJ 1985 Behaviour therapy with obsessive-compulsives: from theory to treatment. In: Mavissakahian M, Turner SM, Michelson L (Eds) Obsessive-Compulsive Disorders: Psychological and Pharmacological Treatments. Plenum, New York

Freeston MH, Ladouceur R, Thibodeau N, Gagnon F 1992 Cognitive intrusions in a non-clinical population II: associations with depressive, anxious and compulsive symptoms. Behaviour Research and Therapy 30: 273–281

Freud S 1895 Obsessions and phobias. In: Strachey J (Ed) 1966 Standard Edition of the Complete Psychological Works of Sigmund Freud 3: 74–82. Hogarth Press, London

1905 Three essays on the theory of sexuality. In: Strachey J (Ed) 1966 Standard Edition of the Complete Psychological Works of Sigmund Freud 7: 123–243. Hogarth Press, London

1907 Obsessive actions and religious practices. In: Strachey J (Ed) 1966 Standard Edition of the Complete Psychological Works of Sigmund Freud 9: 115–128. Hogarth Press, London

1908 Character and anal neuroticism. In: Strachey J (Ed) 1966 Standard Edition of the Complete Psychological Works of Sigmund Freud 9: 169–175. Hogarth Press, London

1909 Notes upon a case of obsessional neurosis. In: Strachey J (Ed) 1966 Standard Edition of the Complete Psychological Works of Sigmund Freud 10: 151–157. Hogarth Press, London

1913a The disposition to obsessional neurosis. In: Strachey J (Ed) 1966 Standard Edition of the Complete Psychological Works of Sigmund Freud 12: 311–326. Hogarth Press, London

1913b Totem and taboo. In: Strachey J (Ed) 1966 Standard Edition of the Complete Psychological Works of Sigmund Freud 13: 1–62. Hogarth Press, London

Frost RO, Lajart CM, Dugus KM, Sher KJ 1988 Information processing among non-clinical compulsives. Behaviour Research and Therapy, 26. 275–277

Fuller S 1985 Styles of Information Processing by Obsessive-Compulsives: Responses to Feared and Neutral Concepts. Unpublished MPhil Thesis, University of Liverpool

Garety PA 1985 Delusions: problems in definition and measurement. British Journal of Medical Psychology 58: 25–34

Garety PA, Everitt BS, Hemsley DR 1988 The characteristics of delusions: a cluster analysis of deluded subjects. European Archives of Psychiatry and Neurological Sciences 237: 112–114

Garety PA, Hemsley DR 1987 Characteristics of delusional experience. European Archives of Psychiatry and Neurological Sciences 236: 294–298

Garety PA, Hemsley DR, Wessely S 1991 Reasoning in deluded, schizophrenic and paranoid patients: biases in performance on a probabilistic inference task. The Journal of Nervous and Mental Disease 179: 194–201

Gholson B, Barker P 1985 Kuhn, Lakatos and Lauden – applications in the history and philosophy of physics and psychology. American Psychologist 40: 755–769

Gittleson NL 1966 The fate of obsessions in depressive psychosis. British Journal of Psychiatry 112: 705–708

Gray JA 1970 The psychophysiological basis of introversion-extraversion. Behaviour Research and Therapy 8: 249–266

1979 Commentary on Eysenck's "The conditioning model of neurosis". Behavioural and Brain Sciences 2: 169–171

1982 The neuropsychology of anxiety. Oxford University Press, London

Green RC, Pitman RK 1986 Tourette Syndrome and Obsessive-Compulsive Disorder. In: Jenike MA, Baer L, Minichiello WE (Eds) Obsessive-Compulsive Disorders: Theory and Management. PSG Publishing Co Inc., Littleton, Mass.

Grünbaum A 1986 Precis of "The Foundations of Psychoanalysis: A Philosophical Critique". Behaviour and Brain Sciences 9: 217–284

Hare E, Price J, Slater E 1972 Fertility in obsessional neurosis. British Journal of Psychiatry 121: 197–205

Hare RM 1981 Moral Thinking. Oxford University Press, Oxford

Havens LL 1966 Pierre Janet. Journal of Nervous and Mental Diseases 143: 383–398

Headland K, McDonald R 1987 Rapid audio-tape treatment of obsessional ruminations. A Case Report. Behavioural Psychotherapy 15: 188–192

Hodgson RJ, Rachman SJ 1972 The effects of contamination and washing in obsessional patients. Behaviour Research and Therapy 10: 111–11

1977 Obsessive-compulsive complaints. Behaviour Research and Therapy 15: 389–395

Hodgson RJ, Rachman SJ, Marks IM 1972 The treatment of chronic obsessive-compulsive neurosis: follow-up and further findings. Behaviour Research and Therapy 10: 181–184

Hole RW, Rush AJ, Beck AT 1979 A cognitive investigation of schizophrenic delusions. Psychiatry 42: 312–319

Hollander E, Schiffman E, Cohen B, Rivera-Stein MA, Rosen W, Gorman JM 1990 Signs of central nervous system dysfunction in obsessive-compulsive disorder. Archives of General Psychiatry 47: 27–32

Huq SF, Garety PA, Hemsley DR 1988 Probabilistic judgments in deluded and non deluded subjects. Quaterly Journal of Experimental Psychology 40A: 801–812

Hymas N, Lees A, Bolton D, Epps K, Head D 1991 The neurology of obsessional slowness. Brain 114: 2203–2233

Ingram IM 1961 Obsessional illness in mental hospital patients. Journal of Mental Science 197: 382–402

Insel TR 1982 Obsessive-compulsive disorder: five clinical questions and a suggested approach. Comprehensive Psychiatry 23: 241–251

Insel TR (Ed) 1984 New Findings in Obsessive-Compulsive Disorder. American Psychiatric Press, Washington

Insel TR 1984 Obsessive-compulsive disorder: the clinical picture. In: Insel TR (Ed) New Findings in Obsessive-Compulsive Disorder. American Psychiatric Press, Washington

1988 Obsessive-compulsive disorder: a neuroethological perspective. Psychopharmacology Bulletin 24: 380–384

1990 Phenomenology of obsessive-compulsive disorder. Journal of Clinical Psychiatry 51: supp. 4.8, discussion 9

Insel TR, Hamilton JA, Guttmacher MB, Murphy DL 1983 d-Amphetamine in obsessive-compulsive disorder. Psychopharmacology 80: 231–235

Jakes IC 1987 The Responses of Different Subgroups of Obsessive-Compulsive Ritualisers to Behaviour Therapy. Unpublished M.Phil Thesis, University of London

1989a Salkovskis on obsessional-compulsive neurosis: a critique. Behaviour Research and Therapy 27: 673–675

1989b Salkovskis on obsessional-compulsive neurosis: a rejoinder. Behaviour Research and Therapy 27: 683–684

1992 An Experimental Investigation of Obsessive-Compulsive Disorder. Unpublished PhD Thesis, University of London.

Janet P 1903 Les Obsessions et la Psychiasthenie, Vol 1. Alcan, Paris (reprinted in Arno, New York, 1976)

Jaspers K 1963 General Psychopathology. Manchester University Press, Manchester

Jenike MA 1984 Obsessive-compulsive disorder: a question of a neurological lesion. Comprehensive Psychiatry 25: 298–304

Jenike MA, Baer l, Minichiello WO (Eds) 1990 Obsessive-Compulsive Disorders: Theory and Management, 2nd edition. Year Book Medical Publishers, Chicago

Karno M, Golding JM, Sorenson SB et al 1988 The epidemilogy of obsessive-compulsive disorder in five US communities. Archives of General Psychiatry 45: 1094–1099

Kendler KS, Glazer WM, Morgenstern H 1983 Dimensions of delusional experiences. American Journal of Psychiatry 140: 466–469

Kettl PA, Marks IM 1986 Neurological factors in obsessive-compulsive disorder: two case reports and a review of the literature. British Journal of Psychiatry 149: 315–319

Kuhn TS 1962 The Structure of Scientific Revolutions. University of Chicago Press, Chicago

Lakatos I 1970 Falsification and the methodology of scientific research progress. In: Lakatos I, Musgrave A (Eds) Criticism and the Growth of Knowledge. Cambridge University Press, Cambridge

Lauden L 1977 Progress and Its Problems. University of California Press, Berkeley

Lewis AJ 1934 Melancholia: a clinical survey of depressive states. Journal of Mental Science 80: 277–318

1936 Problems of obsessional illness. Proceedings of Royal Society of Medicine, 29: 325–336

Lovell K, Noshirvani H, O'Sullivan G, Marks IM 1991 Exposure to audiotaped obsessions vs neutral material: a pilot controlled study of ruminations. Unpublished paper

Luxenberg JS, Flament M, Swedo S, Rapoport JL, Rapoport S 1986 Neuroanatomic abnormalities in obsessive-compulsive disorder detected in quantitative x-ray computed tomography. American Journal of Psychiatry 145: 1089–1094

Makhlouf-Norris F, Jones HG, Norris H 1970 Articulation of conceptual structure in obsessional neurosis. British Journal of Social and Clinical Psychology 9: 264–274

Malan DH 1976 Toward the Validation of Dynamic Psychotherapy. Plenum, New York 1979 Individual Psychotherapy and the Science of Psychodynamics. Butterworths, London

Marks IM 1981 Cure and Care of Neuroses. Wiley, Chichester

Marks IM, Stern RS, Mawson D, Cobb J, McDonald R 1980 Clomipramine and exposure for obsessive-compulsive rituals, I and II. British Journal of Psychiatry 136: 1–25

McFall ME, Wollersheim JP 1979 Obsessive-compulsive neurosis: a cognitive-behavioral formulation and approach to treatment. Cognitive Therapy and Research 3: 333–348

McKeon J, Roa B, Mann A 1984 Life events and personality trait in obsessive-compulsive neurosis. British Journal of Psychiatry 144: 185–189

Melden AL 1961 Free Action. Routledge and Kegan Paul, London

Miller DG 1980 A repertory grid study of obsessionality: distinctive cognitive structure or distinctive cognitive content? British Journal of Medical Psychology 53: 59–66

Minneka S 1986 The frightful complexity of the origins of fears. Paper presented at the British Psychological Society Annual Conference, Sheffield

Mishkin M, Malamut B, Bachevalier J 1984 Memories and habits: two neural systems. In: Lynch G, McGaugh JL, Weinberger NM (Eds) Neurobiology of Learning and Memory. Guildford Press, New York

Montgomery S 1990 OCD and 5-HT re-uptake inhibitors. Paper presented at the Duphar National Symposium on Obsessive-Compulsive Disorder, London

Mowrer OH 1939 A stimuli-response theory of anxiety. Psychological Review 46: 553–565 1960 Learning Theory and Behaviour. Wiley, New York

Mullen P 1979 Phenomenology of disordered mental function. In: Hill P, Murray R, Thorley G (Eds) Essentials of Postgraduate Psychiatry. Academic Press, London

Murray RM, Clifford C, Fulker DW, Smith A 1981 Does heredity contribute to obsessional traits and symptoms? In: Tsuang MT (Ed) Genetic Issues. Academic Press, New York

Myers JK, Weissman MM, Tischler GL et al 1984 Six-month prevalence of psychiatric disorders in three sites. Archives of General Psychiatry 41: 959–971

Pavlov IP 1928 (trans. 1955) Selected Works. Foreign Languages Publishing House, Moscow

Persons JB, Foa EB 1984 Processing of fearful and neutral information by obsessive-compulsives. Behaviour Research and Therapy 22: 259–265

Phillips LD, Edwards W 1966 Conservatism in a simple probabilistic inference task. Journal of Experimental Psychology 72: 346–354

Pitman RK 1983 Tourette's syndrome and ethology (letter). American Journal of Psychiatry 140: 652 1984 Janet's obsessions and psychasthenia: a synopsis. Psychiatric Quaterly 56: 291–314

1987a Pierre Janet on obsessive-compulsive disorder. Archives of General Psychiatry 44: 226–232

1987b A cybernetic model of obsessive-compulsive psychopathology. Comprehensive Psychiatry 28: 334–343

1989 Animal models of compulsive behaviour. Biological Psychiatry 26: 189–198

Pollack JM 1979 Obsessive-compulsive personality: a review. Psychological Bulletin 86: 225–241

1987 Relationship of obsessive-compulsive personality to obsessive-compulsive disorder: a review of the literature. The Journal of Psychology 121(2): 137–148

Popper K 1963 Conjectures and Refutations. Routledge and Kegan Paul, London

1972 The Logic of Scientific Discovery. Hutchinson, London

Putnam H 1974 The "corroboration" of theories. In: Honderich T, Burnyeat M 1979 Philosophy as It Is. Penguin Books, Harmondsworth

Rachman SJ 1974 Primary obsessional slowness. Behaviour Research and Therapy 12: 9–18

1978 An analysis of obsessions. Behavioural Analysis and Modification 2: 253–278

1980 Emotional processing. Behaviour Research and Therapy 18: 51–60

1993 Obsessions, responsibility and guilt. Behaviour Research and Therapy 31: 149–154

Rachman SJ, Hodgson R, Marks IM 1971 The treatment of chronic obsessive-compulsive neurosis. Behaviour Research and Therapy 9: 237–247

1973 The treatment of obsessive-compulsive neurotics by modelling and flooding. Behaviour Research and Therapy 11: 463–471

Rachman SJ, Hodgson RJ 1980 Obsessions and Compulsions. Prentice Hall, Englewood Cliffs

Rachman SJ, Parkinson L 1981 Unwanted intrusive cognitions. Advances in Behaviour Research and Therapy 3: 89–123

Rachman SJ, de Silva P, Roper G 1976 The spontaneous decay of compulsive urges. Behaviour Research and Therapy 14: 445–453

Rachman SJ, de Silva P 1978 Abnormal and normal obsessions. Behaviour Research and Therapy 16: 233–248

Rapoport JL 1989 The biology of obsessions and compulsions. Scientific American (March): 62–69

Rapoport JL, Wise SP 1988 Obsessive-compulsive disorder: evidence for basal ganglia dysfunction. Psychopharmacology Bulletin 24: 380–384

Rasmussen SA, Eisen JL 1990 Epidemiology of obsessive compulsive disorder. Journal of Clinical Psychiatry 51:2(Suppl): 10–14

Rasmussen SA, Tsuang MT 1986 Epidemiology and clinical features of obsessive-compulsive disorder. In: Jenike MA, Baer L, Minichiello WE (Eds) Obsessive-Compulsive Disorders: Theory and Management. PSG Publishing Co Inc, Littleton, Mass.

Raven JC 1965 Guide to Using the Mill Hill Vocabulary Scale with the Progressive Matrices Scale. Lewis, London

Reed GF 1968 Some formal qualities of obsessional thinking. Psychiatria Clinica 1: 382–392

1969a "Under-inclusion" – a characteristic of obsessional personality disorder:1. British Journal of Psychiatry 115: 781–785

1969b "Under-inclusion" – a characteristic of obsessional personality disorder: 2. British Journal of Psychiatry 115: 787–790

1976 Indecisiveness in obsessional-compulsive disorder. British Journal of Social and Clinical Psychology 15: 443–445

1977a Obsessional personality disorder and remembering. British Journal of Psychiatry 130: 177–83

1977b Obsessional cognition: performance on two numerical tests. British Journal of Psychiatry 130: 184–185

1985 Obsessional Experience and Compulsive Behaviour: A Cognitive Structural Approach. Academic Press, London

1991 The cognitive characteristics of obsessional disorder. In: Magaro P (Ed) Cognitive Bases of Mental Disorders. Annual Review of Psychopathology, Vol 1. Sage Publications, Newburg Park

Robins LN, Helzer JG, Groughnan J et al 1981 National Instiute of Mental Health Diagnostic Interview Schedule: Its history, characteristics, and validity. Archives of General Psychiatry 38: 381–384

Roper G, Rachman SJ, Marks IM 1975 Passive and participant modelling in exposure treatment of obsessive-compulsive neurotics. Behaviour Research and Therapy 13: 271–279

Ryle G 1949 The Concept of Mind. Hutchinson, London

Salkovskis PM 1985 Obsessive-compulsive problems: a cognitive behavioural analysis. Behaviour Research and Therapy 23: 571–583

1989 Cognitive-behavioural factors and the persistence of intrusive thoughts in obsessional problems. Behaviour Research and Therapy 27: 677–682

Salkovskis PM, Westbrook D 1989 Behaviour therapy and obsessional ruminations: can failure be turned into success? Behaviour Research and Therapy 27: 149–160

Sandler J, Hazari A 1960 The "obsessional": on the psychological classification of obsessional character traits and symptoms. British Journal of Medical Psychology 33: 113–122

Schneider K 1925 (trans 1958) Psychopathic Personalities. Trans. Hamilton JW. Cassell, London

Seligman MEP 1971 Phobias and preparedness. Behavior Therapy 2: 307–320

de Silva P 1988 Obsessive-compulsive disorder. In: Miller E and Cooper PJ (Eds) Adult Abnormal Psychology. Churchill Livingstone, London

de Silva P, Rachman SJ, Seligman M 1977 Prepared phobias and obsessions: therapeutic outcome. Behaviour Research and Therapy 15: 54–77

Snaith P 1981 Clinical Neurosis. Oxford University Press, London

Southworth S, Kirsch I 1988 The role of expectancy in exposure-generated fear reduction in agoraphobia. Behaviour Research and Therapy 26: 113–120

Stengel E 1945 A study on some clinical aspects of the relationship between obsessional neurosis and psychotic reaction types. Journal of Mental Science 91: 166–187

Stern RS, Cobb JP (1978) Phenomenology of obsessive-compulsive neurosis. British Journal of Psychiatry 132: 233–239

Strauss JS 1969 Hallucinations and delusions as points on continua function. Archives of General Psychiatry 20: 581–586

Symington N 1986 The Analytic Experience: Lectures from the Tavistock. Free Association Books, London

Teasdale J 1974 Learning models of obsessive-compulsive disorder. In: Beech HR (Ed) Obsessional States. Methuen, London

Turner SM, Beidel DC, Nathan RS 1985 Biological factors in obsessive-compulsive disorder. Psychological Bulletin 97: 430–450

Volans PJ Styles of Probabilistic Inference in Obsessional and Phobic Patients. Unpublished MPhil Thesis, University of London

1976 Styles of decision making and probability appraisal in selected obsessional and phobic patients. British Journal of Social and Clinical Psychology 15: 305–317

Walker VJ 1973 Explanations in obsessional neurosis. British Journal of Psychiatry 123: 675–680

Wittgenstein L 1953 Philosophical Investigations. Basil Blackwell, Oxford

Wolpe J 1958 Psychotherapy by Reciprocal Inhibition. Stanford University Press, Stanford

Woodfield A 1976 Teleology. Cambridge University Press, Cambridge

Zohar J, Insel TR, Zohar-Kadouch RC, Hill JL, Murphy DL 1988 Serotonergic responsivity in obsessive-compulsive disorder: effects of chronic clomipramine treatment. Archives of General Psychiatry 45: 167–172

Zohar J, Mueller EA, Insel TR, Zohar-Kadouch RC, Murphy DL 1987 Serotonergic responsivity in obsessive-compulsive disorder: comparison of patients and healthy controls. Archives of General Psychiatry 44: 946–951

Author index

Subject index